Collana Universitaria Athena

o8

Bianca Buchal

Maternity Awareness

Expecting Mindfully: A Conscious Guide to Motherhood

Translated by Caterina Coluccia Civelli

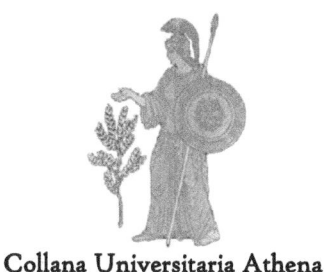

Collana Universitaria Athena

Stella Mattutina Edizioni

Collection | **Collana Universitaria Athena**
UA 08

Title | Maternity Awareness
Author | Bianca Buchal
Translation | Caterina Coluccia Civelli
Cover | Stella Mattutina Edizioni®
Immagine in copertina | Getty Images
ISBN | 9788899462468

© All rights reserved
Copyright © 2018 Stella Mattutina Edizioni
No part of this book can be reproduced
without the consent of the Author and Editor

Original Title: Gravidanza consapevole

Stella Mattutina Edizioni®
Via del Lago n. 26; 50018, Scandicci (Fi) - Italy
Tel./Fax +39/055.769044; 3402418469
Web: www.stellamattutinaedizioni.com
e-mail: stellamattutinaedizioni@gmail.com

*Special thanks
to my friend Evelyn Disseau
and to the midwife Mara Pagani
for their precious ideas and suggestions*

Index

Introduction 11
I. The Woman, Mother of Humanity 13
II. The Father 17
III. The conception 21
IV. The bonding 26
V. Parenthood 30
VI. Communicating with your child's soul 34
VII. The pregnancy 38
VIII. Gestation from the medical point of view 44
IX. Blessing ritual of an expectant mother 47
X. The sound 49
XI. Let us go to the music world 53
XII. …and let's dress our life with colors 55
XIII. Centres for the accompanying towards pregnancy
    and childbirth 59
XIV. Let's talk about nutrition 62
XV. Smoking and alcohol during pregnancy 66
XVI. The mother's stress on the quality of fetal life 68
XVII. Some advice for a conscious, positive and happy
    pregnancy 70
XVIII. The massage 72
XIX. A child speaks to his parents from the womb 75
XX. The choice of the clinic 81
XXI. My childbirth: a magical event 85
XXII. Ode to birth 89

xxiii. The pain of labour......................93
xxiv. Caesarean section......................95
xxv. Childbirth in water 99
xxvi. Labour and childbirth 103
xxvii. "Obstetrician" and Midwife..............107
xxviii. Lotus Birth..........................109
xxix. Welcoming the child at birth..............115
xxx. The wound that medicine does not recognise......123
xxxi. Possible disorders during pregnancy.............127
xxxii. Post-partum depression 133
xxxiii. The breastfeeding 139
xxxiv. The weaning..........................143
xxxv. How to carry a child on yourself 147
xxxvi. Education............................149
xxxvii. The mystery, the creation, the sacredness 153
xxxviii. Conclusion 155
xxxix. The love 164
xl. Conclusive reflections 165
Appendix 1 170
Appendix 2 172
Appendix 3 174
Appendix 4 177
The Author 180

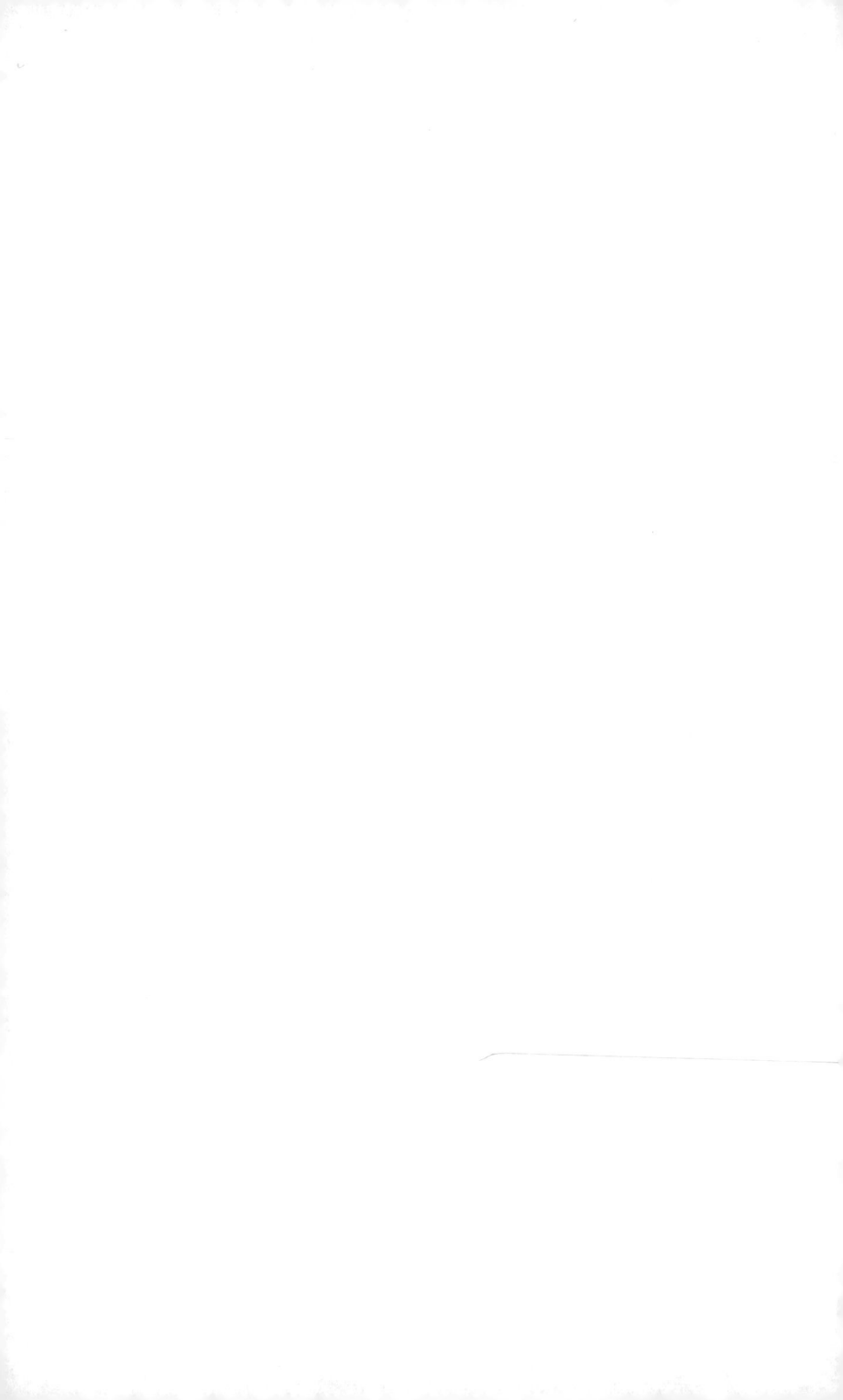

Introduction

In this book, I especially address you, Woman. I would like to pass on the basics to best fulfil your role as a Mother, enhancing all your wonderful potential. But I also turn to you, Man, so that you may become aware of the particularly important role that you will be called to play, the moment you become aware that you will become a Father.

From the content of these pages you can easily guess with how much joy and contentment I turn to Women, to help them find their rightful place in the family and in society, as well as in the role entrusted to them by Nature: to be a Mother.

By this I do not mean to say that the role of Mother is exclusively that of giving birth to children. No! The maternal feeling, so exquisitely feminine, can express itself in many forms: towards everyone and everything around us.

I believe it is extremely important to transmit to you, future Mothers, basic and useful information, enriched by those values that have long since been shelved, so you can proceed in all serenity towards a happy motherhood, fully aware of the importance of your task.

Such information will not only serve to eradicate those fears and senses of inadequacy that often arise in the face of such a great undertaking as to giving birth to a new creature, but above all to understand the meaning of giving human society a new being, an individual who will have received from you the best, necessary imprints and examples to be able to positively carry out the task for which it is born.

It will be good that even young people of any age receive these notions, to have clear ideas when it is time for them to form a family. You will then understand the meaning of the subtitle: *The woman's task: build a better world.*

With friendship, from your
Bianca

I

The Woman, Mother of Humanity

Women should become conscious of their role and feel that they are the Mothers of humanity, because only they have been given the ability to bring new life into the world. And, depending on the physical and psychological effort they dedicate to this function, tomorrow's Humanity will develop and rely upon this. They have a great responsibility towards society, a responsibility that must obviously be shared by men who, though in a different role, play an integral and important part.

The role that nature has given women is so immense that not taking it fully into consideration would seem offensive to the magnificent force that governs this extraordinary event.

Let's start from the beginning. Just as the light comes on when we flick the switch, so life springs forth when the sperm meets the ovum. Each one without the other can do nothing. Together they produce light, life. From that moment onwards, the woman offers her body as a container. Thus, thanks to all the elements and conditions she makes available, all products of nature just as she is a product of nature herself, the ancient matrix that has, since the beginning of time and with infallible intelligence produced millions and millions of creatures, can start its creative work.

Women, in this role, become partners with the Creator, that indescribable power that is the very one that has created all that we behold. One only has to look up at the night sky to be amazed by the sight of the celestial bodies set out in a pre-established order. In a cosmic order that regulates everything, always respecting perfect harmony. This is how the creation of the tiny body of the baby comes about, where every cell knows what function it belongs to, exactly, in a cosmic order. Everything responds exactly to the Law of Evolution, as we can see that over time, very slowly, everything evolves, everything is perfected.

Naturally, a human being is not just a physical organism, but has intellect, a soul and a spirit that allow it to show intelligence and sensibility at various levels. Therefore, a woman, in the way she performs this role, both physically and spiritually, must respect this situation of harmony, allowing the being that is taking shape inside her to take advantage of this fundamental state of well-being, so as to obtain the best result possible, both physically and psychologically.

At the core of this Harmony, naturally, lies Love.

Everything is Love.

If during the pregnancy, we give love to the little ones, we talk to them about beautiful things, we sing for them and make them grow with the joy of being waited for, a new generation that will bring peace on earth will be born. It will just be necessary to give birth to our children with love, conceive them and soak them with love. If all the children will be born drenched with love, during their growth, Love will become part of their nature. This will be transformed into mutual respect, tolerance, and all those qualities that we lack at present and that will enable peaceful coexistence.

<u>Peace begins in the mother's womb.</u> This was said by both Gandhi and many other philosophers. *The secret to improving the future of humanity is found right in life before birth.* For almost half a century, many scientists and researchers, thanks to tools made possible by biotechnology, have begun to probe the intrauterine world and this is how it was possible to know the true identity of the child in the uterus.

Once it was believed that the gestating baby was just a mass of totally insensitive cells. Today, however, we know for sure that the child lives in symbiosis with his mother by participating in every thought, every feeling and behaviour. Therefore, the mother must set her way of life according to the task she is carrying out: <u>*the creation of a new individual, who will have to bring only positive things into the world.*</u> *The mother is able to perform miracles, since it is she who holds the key to the forces of life*, while her father and the surrounding environment play an important role.

This is how a renewed humanity can be forged.

Of course, all this is, at least for now, is only a dream, but if you fully understand the sense of what was said above, that *woman is the Mother of humanity*, then everything could really change!

The task of Mothers continues, after giving birth, with education to respect, to righteousness, to Good in general.

Only then will the men look at their women through other eyes and see in them as creatures that deserve all the trust, collaboration and support. Once this point of view is accepted, it is important to spread it by transmitting what you believe in, to the daughters, to the sisters, to the friends, but also to the men of the family.

Can you imagine what it would be like to have a world where only children born to love were born? Would it not be a wonderful thing? This depends only on the woman, naturally supported by her partner, *who must recognise her role as Mother of humanity*. This is also said by a well-known French gynaecologist, Michel Odent: "*Society will never change if we do not change the way we give birth to our children*".

II

The Father

In the past, studies on parental behaviour during prenatal life focused on the mothers' behaviour. Nobody cared about the behaviour of the fathers. Starting to introduce oneself in this field, has represented a very important step.

Now we meet young fathers who denote a protective and loving behaviour towards their pregnant woman. They are those fathers who are waiting to welcome their child with open arms, those who speak with the child, who sing for him and caress him through the belly, who listen to the beating of his little heart. Those fathers are present and, although they do not realise it, they are in communication with the child even when they show love and affection toward their mother. These fathers worry when the mother is fatigued or not well, and they get busy with home chores more than usual.

They accompany the mother to the childbirth preparation course, learn to massage their woman and feel involved with a surprising interest, as if they were to give birth themselves. In fact, pregnancy is not exclusive to women and it is right that the couple live the experience together. It is during the pregnancy that the right balance is established within the couple.

The gestation period can cause the woman to experience some difficult moments, both from a physical and psychological perspective. In these cases, the father reacts with a lot of sweetness and a good dose of patience and understanding. During childbirth, he represents an important support for women and most men experience participation positively. During labour, the fathers follow the contractions, breathe together with the woman and above all, act as a continuous and loving encouragement. It is during this period that the roles of each one become evident, especially the role of the father, a role that for too long has been denied.

In order to instil the new paternal image into oneself and to perform this function well, it is advisable that a strong bond is created within the triad, from the very first moment of gestation. While in the past men did not have access to the intrauterine world, they are now able to activate a deep and satisfying relationship with their children long before their birth, much to the delight of their mother and child.

Today, the desire for paternity is often more linked to unconscious feelings, dreams and fantasies. The child that a man desires and wishes for is a child that is the best version of himself – what he would have liked to become and was not able to. A child to whom he would give everything he wanted to have and that he never had. This makes a man more inclined to collect messages and unconscious fantasies, linked to a dream of paternity that is more emotional than social.

At the time of birth, the fathers declare that they have lived such an experience with such intensity and happiness that they would never have imagined being able to feel.

These are the fathers of the new generation.

Fathers who know how to get off their pedestal to live in harmony with their woman and child. *Fathers who can answer in the truest way to the needs of their children,* at any age, and that represent an important reference point.

This new father is more in touch with everyday experiences, also because today *he is more capable than ever to accept and make use of the "feminine" elements of his personality, such as tenderness.* However, in order to be able to carry out this role as a parent, there is no better way to know one's child than to have lovingly followed him from conception.

It is a completely new transformation, that is still in progress.

There is also a *greater ability of the man to share that mysterious event, that the woman lives within herself through pregnancy.* He shows this in many ways, through the tenderness of physical contact, physical proximity that is not only sexual, like when he caresses the belly and approaches his ear in order to hear the baby's heartbeat. The father takes part in the happiness, the satisfaction and in the pride of the woman for the child who grows inside her but also in her anxieties and her concerns. He accompanies her to the gynaecologist, to childbirth preparation courses and chooses with her the clothing, the cradle, the name... She feels less distant from the child also by being able to see the ultrasound.

If the new dad follows with such participation the evolution of his son even before birth, he will undoubtedly continue to do so even after, accompanying him step by step during childhood, adolescence and beyond, until the child has acquired, within the family, solid foundations to take flight and become independent, self-sufficient and live his life. In fact, the father, as the third pole of the family triangle, is the male element that when the time comes, will favour the separation of the child from the mother, projecting it towards the world.

However, the family will remain an important reference point for the child. A child raised in a healthy environment – in which he is listened to, understood and in which he can express himself – will never feel the need to join a "flock" to find company.

It is in the spirit of the gift, not of exchange, *that the father will carry out his educational function*, without expecting any reward. If this happens, it will come when the child has grown up.

III

The conception

Bringing a child into the world is not a decision that can be taken lightly. The pace of our day, our uncertainties, our fears, our needs, everything requires us to carefully reflect upon this choice and it is right. In fact, the presence of a child will absorb our attention for many years and we must be willing to give up many moments of the day that normally satisfy us. In addressing the arrival of a child, *one must prepare oneself to completely change one's lifestyle in order to adapt and prepare to the new task. However,* on the other hand, *we are faced with such a great joy, capable of withdrawing the discomfort of every renunciation.*

In order to be able to make a fair and impartial assessment, potential future parents should be adequately informed about all the positive and joyful aspects, but also about the most challenging aspects of having a child. They should also know the importance of the relationship with the child not only after birth, but also during gestation, a decisive period in the life of every individual in which all future existence is reflected.

Nowadays, there are now many couples who, to face a task as important as that of becoming parents, try to refine their sensitivity and increase their skills by preparing in advance for this task.

Among many other things, it is useful that they are aware that, as physics teaches, every cell possesses certain characteristics, by multiplying itself, transmits the same qualities to the new cells. Therefore, if the initial cell is impregnated with strong vibrations of Love, so will all the others. Thus, a child conceived with Love will be born. In fact, *Love is food, it is life for the child in it's shaping.*

Every child should be born in the name of Love, *only if truly desired.* Unwanted children should no longer come into the world.

Just like the farmer who, to obtain a good harvest, ploughs the land of his field, cleans it up of stones and weeds, then fertilises it and, when everything is ready, before throwing the seed, takes care that this is fresh and healthy, so should the future parents: prepare the best soil on which to give birth to a new life. This does not only mean controlling one's state of health, but also resolving tensions and old grudges towards parents, relatives and friends, to meet parenting without old weights that often weigh down existence.

A son? Yes, but when you are sure you can give him everything he needs. Affective stability, economic security, time and space are certainties that we try to reach before giving birth to a child. This is precisely the factor that contributes to giving rise to a more conscious motherhood and paternity. Today, it is increasingly rare for a child to be a child of chance, however, he is increasingly a child of desire. Contraception, widespread since the 1970s, has changed the way of becoming parents. A child should still be conceived when a strong and deep understanding has been established between the two partners *and born when one really wants it,* not when it "arrives", as it occurred in the past.

However, the desire of having a child cannot always be subject to the logic of reason. It is something very strong, instinctive, "passionate", which also comes from the regions of the unconscious, which sometimes breaks into the bond of a couple, perhaps at the least appropriate time. The important thing, however, is to be able to give space to the unexpected and accept that something not completely programmed occurs.

Once conception has taken place, experiencing pregnancy with an anxious behaviour of getting to know your child, would imply the loss of a unique opportunity to savour the nine-month period that is one of the most beautiful moments, in terms of dialogue and affection not only in the relationship with the child, but also between the future parents.

Making love

When we talk about making love, we focus on the pleasure we experience, but when it comes to procreating, making love becomes a much more challenging thing. In fact, consciously conceiving means to unite in love to procreate another human being. We must not forget that this process is miraculous. In various parts of the world there are communities in which the sexual act made with the intention of procreating is accompanied by songs, prayers and rituals, in order to encourage the union of the egg and spermatozoa invoking divine intervention. Whether or not you believe in supernatural power, it is certain that when a new life begins in the womb, we must admit that it is an extraordinary process.

In modern life, the sacred rituals that accompany a conscious conception or a joyful birth have been forgotten. Don't you think it's time to restore them? It is however necessary to ensure that the right conditions are present: physical, emotional, psychological and spiritual.

*Two beings that unite
to conceive a child
they must act in the light
and in the awareness of working together
to achieve a marvellous endeavour.*

Omraam Mikhaël Aïvanhov

IV

The bonding

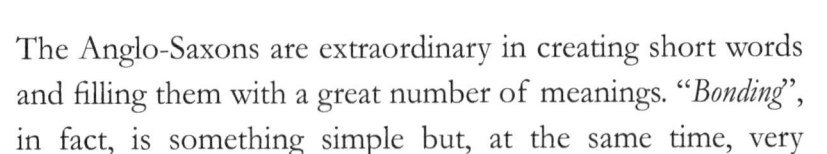

The Anglo-Saxons are extraordinary in creating short words and filling them with a great number of meanings. *"Bonding"*, in fact, is something simple but, at the same time, very complex. A word born in the early seventies, bonding means "to glue, to connect, to cement".

For those who might not remember, the great ethologist Konrad Lorenz, who conducted experiments on geese, the geese followed him everywhere because, at the time of their birth, the Viennese ethologist was recognised as "parent" and was able to establish with them the imprinting. We, on the other hand, are interested in bonding that, unlike imprinting, is a process of forming the unique bond between parents and children that starts from conception, which manifests itself in a concrete form throughout pregnancy and that continues in different forms also after.

It is a profound and lasting relationship, based on the bi-directional Love that exists between parent and child. It is a delicate, complicated and complex process, whose effectiveness can vary between men, according to the way in which it occurs. Bonding creates a specific and permanent connection that is established in that period of time, when parents live a moment of strong emotionality, favouring a great communicative sensitivity that produces effective responses to the needs of the child.

At the beginning of the pregnancy, the bonding is mainly cultivated by the mother, who can accompany the growth of the creature that is forming in it with appropriate stimulations, caresses and positive thoughts, in order to enrich its growth with an array of psychological aspects that, later, they will prove invaluable. At birth, in the two hours after giving birth, *the ideal would be to put the newborn in the arms of the mother, skin against skin, keeping the umbilical cord intact,* if the health of mother and child allow it and especially if the protocol of the clinic contemplates it! In fact, the child experiences a quiet waking period, where he can open his eyes, look and recognise his parents, listen to voices and sounds, search for (alone) the mother's breast, recover through the tender embrace of his mother and feel protected and reassured.

At this stage, the focus is very high and we could say that for the child…the first impression is what matters. It is precisely here that the process commences in a more consistent form. We should avoid first impressions to happen far from the mother, from her body, from her voice, from her warmth, from her loving touch and naturally involving also the father.

Two hours after the meeting with mum and dad, the child slips into a phase of drowsiness: he has to regain his strength and often during this period, he is subjected to normal health checks. At this point the reception on behalf of the parents has already happened, so bonding is consolidated.

If we understand the importance of bonding, we also understand the seriousness of failing to receive the child. Recently, many study groups have carried out analyses on the behavioural characteristics of children who were received with care and method. The results, needless to say, are more than encouraging. I further explore this fundamental point in the chapter "*Receiving the child at birth*".

It is always the environment that shapes the child: the behaviour of the parents, their warmth, their state of mind, their love.

In a remote region of East Africa, the customs of an ethnic group and its magical world are told where the future Mother is seen as lead role.

She knows the birth day of her baby even before it is conceived because the baby is born first of all in the Mother's mind. When she wishes to conceive a child, the woman goes to the forest, sits at the foot of a tree and waits to hear the song of the child that will be born from her.

The wise of that community say that this is the true moment of conception. Later, the Mother will return to the village and teach that song to the Father.

Through Love the child is called.

All the women of the tribe will have to learn that melody, so that in labour and at the moment of birth the child is welcomed into this world by the singing of his own melody. The same song will be sung during every illness, on special occasions and in every ritual of growth and development. At the end of life, the most loved people will gather around the deathbed and sing that song for the last time.

Jack Kornfield

V

Parenthood

The mother and the father both weave fantasies around the child that will come, everything is still to be invented. This inner process is very important when becoming a parent. In this way, an "affective" mental space is also prepared, in which to welcome the little guest.

The man projects on his son, even before he is born, a future reality, with precise contours, like the behaviours and projects that will bind him to his son. It is therefore an extremely active and concrete way of imagining the child and the relationship with him based on "doing together".

On the other hand, the woman tends to imagine the child still as a part of herself, within her body and mind. If, you imagine it already born, it is still a very small child, to be held in the arms, to be nourished, covered, warmed up, cuddled...

During the pregnancy, it is good not to consolidate your desire that a boy is born rather than a girl. If a girl is born while the parents wanted so much a boy, the child will perceive that she is not the child that the parents wanted, and this feeling could disturb her existence.

As long as the parents' imagination expresses itself in a very wide range of possibilities, the child's future remains open, not affected by their desires. If you leave space for it, it will then be the child himself who, little by little, wants to be accepted for what he is, and not for what he could have been: a boy or a girl.

However, it should not be forgotten that even if during pregnancy mother and child form a single body, in fact they are two distinct persons, each with their own destiny and their own plan for life. The child is born free.

Building limits for those born free is a crime.

As long as the child is small, ingenuous and led to believe in everyone, it is easy for him to find himself in the web of constraints, but then, as he becomes aware, he feels that he lacks oxygen, light and vital space it needs to grow. That's how the unhappiness and loss of self-esteem is born, leading to the reversal of the march. The uphill road becomes a downhill path, a makeshift journey, a path to the opposite, a surrender, an obscure retreat. Faced with a disparity of strength, the child adapts to ensure survival. However, this forced acceptance is the seed of rebellion, of power and violence. In fact, a misunderstanding can slow down growth more than the lack of a meal. To grow, it takes above all Love. The lack of Love, of joy, of harmony with oneself and with others inevitably leads to illness and to the breaking of one's equilibrium.

The poet Kahlil Gibran, in his book The Prophet, writes:
Your children do not belong to you. They are the children of the appeal that Life does to itself. You put them in the

world but you do not create them. They live with you but they are not yours. You can give them your love, but not your thoughts, because they have their own ideas. You can provide a dwelling place for their bodies, but not for their souls, for they live in the house of tomorrow where you cannot enter, not even in a dream. You can force yourself to be like them, but do not try to make them similar to you, because life does not come back and does not stop yesterday. You are the bows with which your children are launched into the world as living arrows.

*The unleashing of the atom's power
has changed everything
except our way of thinking.
Now, if humanity wants to survive,
it must resort to an essentially
new way of thinking.*

Albert Einstein

VI

Communicating with your child's soul

Let us now read the description of a wonderful guided meditation for future parents from the book *Welcoming the Soul of the Child*, by Jill Hopkins:

> In any place and in any difficult situation a mother finds herself, she is hosting within herself the most extraordinary of processes. She must then give herself five minutes a day to formulate positive thoughts, to listen to the favourite piece of music or to feed her soul in the way she likes: her sweetness will increase enormously until becoming an integral part of her, for all the future years. Five minutes of attention are worth years of inner well-being. In the imaginary that follows, you, future mother, and you, future father, will be led to meet your child and to dialogue with it. If you decide to do this work together, remember not to exchange any suggestions.
>
> During this meditation silence is essential. It will be a special dialogue, because the unborn child, despite being a human being, does not yet belong to your world and knows nothing of your reality. It will be like a dialogue with a being from another planet, living in conditions completely different from yours.
>
> However, this creature is infinitely close to you, it is part of you. For now, his destiny is your destiny, his body is your body, and that is why you can have a subtle communication with the child. The only way to make the dialogue possible

is to become receptive, just as receptive as your child will be and to listen to deeply, consciously, openly. Now close your eyes, relax for a few minutes and follow the rhythm of your breathing. Do not force it, but make it slower and deeper. By paying attention to your breathing, you will become more prone to sensations.

Now put aside your daily worries, your opinions, your habits, even your needs. Let your breath go on alone. You are a silent consciousness. As a silent presence, you realise that your awareness is becoming wider and deeper: bare awareness, free from any concept, particularly capable of incorporating even the subtlest of sensations, emotions, even the most intimate ones. Immerse yourself in awareness; you can find yourself anywhere: in the depths of the oceans or on the highest peak in the mountains, in the desert, on a beach, in the forest or in a leaf, on a rainbow, in the centre of the earth or on a star. Among all the places that appear in your imagination, choose the mystery where life begins, the enchanted interior where the darkness reigns, where you can meet the child of your dreams.

Now you travel through various layers of tissue until you meet the placenta, through the wonderful geometry of the cells, through amazing landscapes, towards the deep place where life is created.

Now reach the place where your child lives. A little heart beats, a form moves in the amniotic fluid, suspended in space. Your eyes do not yet see the familiar forms, but are open to infinity. You have the impression that there is something powerful and sublime at work, where, with a precise rhythm and a knowledge that goes back to distant times, everything is evolving. You are there with your awareness. You have the feeling of the presence of a creature: it is your child!

Now take the time necessary to make contact with this

presence and be very open to any message that may come to you.
Listen to it.
The presence of the unborn child is already a message. Feel your state of mind, its being there.
If you put aside any supposition, you will receive messages with surprising clarity. At this point your child will communicate with you actively. Listen to him! He will tell you where he is from. He will tell you what his wishes, his needs are. He will talk to you about his abilities and the future: as soon as you hear it, be careful not to interfere with your own projections and desires. Now it is up to you to communicate. You can express everything that will please your child, project on him a river of tenderness, the desire to keep it in your arms and the joy of knowing that it exists. You will be able to transmit the images of the most beautiful things in the world in which he will be born. You can communicate with music, with gentle lullabies, with cheerful songs. You can communicate with him in words, whispering sweet expressions. It is up to you how you prefer to communicate with your little one.
You can continue the dialogue for as long as you want or resume it at intervals. In this way, you will create a deep bond: prenatal bonding.

The child learns what he lives

If he lives in rebuke, he will become intransigent.
If he lives in hostility, he will become aggressive.
If he lives in derision, he will become shy.
If he lives in rejection,
he will become a disheartened person.
If he lives in serenity, he will become more balanced.
If he lives in encouragement,
he will become more enterprising.
If he lives in appreciation,
he will become more comprehensive.
If he lives in loyalty, he will become more just.
If he lives in clarity, he will become more assured.
If he lives in esteem, he will become more confident.
If he lives in friendship, he will become a friend for the whole world.

VII

The pregnancy

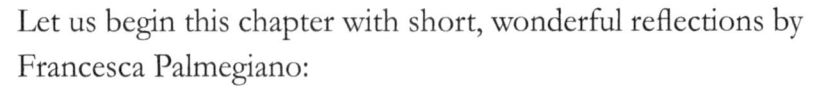

Let us begin this chapter with short, wonderful reflections by Francesca Palmegiano:

> *A thousand feelings and emotions have overwhelmed you when you found out that you were expecting a baby. The adventure of birth begins in this way, amid a whirlwind of amazement, joy and fear... but now relax and enjoy, day by day, the most marvellous of experiences.*
>
> *It is not you who gives life, but it is life that enters you, works in you and does your task. You must be ready to receive it, to cooperate. Ready to give all of you: your body, your mind, your emotions, but also to receive so much when you come into visual contact with the fruit of this energy and you can touch and embrace your little one. Your child is not your property. You have allowed him to enter the world and you will grow it with all your love. You will not do this work only for him but for everyone, because your child is an integral part of the whole universe and if you help him grow healthy and strong in the body, free in the mind and good in his feelings, it will be a harmonious note in the great universal symphony.*

Life before birth is a fascinating theme that involves physical, scientific, psychological, emotional and social factors that were never imagined until a few years ago. In fact, it is now known that the human being is the sum of the experiences already made during intrauterine life, experiences that will have a great impact on the rest of existence.

Every emotion, every mood, but also the interest and effort that the mother puts in any action during the day is reflected on him. It should not be forgotten that everything that the child absorbs during this period remains as an indelible mark in its mind, as a basis for his growth and for the formation of his character. *It is evident and fundamental that parents, aware of the influence they are able to exert on the nascent creature, create in their environment a welcoming and serene atmosphere throughout the pregnancy period.* At the base, there will naturally be demonstrations and expressions of love. *Love is nourishment for the developing child.*

The father is not only responsible for sharing his child's expectation intensely, but for creating an atmosphere of respect, love, support, protection and tranquillity around the mother.

Therefore, pregnancy is not just that period of nine months in which we are eagerly awaiting the "happy event" and during which it is necessary to undergo various medical checks, but much more.

Before beginning a pregnancy, it is good to dissolve deep nodes which, in part, have to do with the fear of pain. It is important to learn not to be afraid, to let go and overcome stiffness and panic. To achieve this, it will be very important to attend a course to accompany pregnancy. It is also necessary *to eliminate the individual traumas sedimented in our mind.* To this end there are many techniques, and each one, will apply the one that is most congenial to him. It will also be good to smooth out old situations of tension with parents, relatives and friends, to give birth to the new creature on a "clean ground". During the gestation period, the baby, immersed in amniotic fluid, is like a switched recorder. Since, from the outset, not only the physical body is formed, but also the child's mind, *everything that succeeds in giving the mother well-being, joy, serenity and balance will certainly benefit the little one too.*

Today, science presents the child to us as a small intelligent, sociable being, in need of affection and eager for dialogue, attention and love, endowed with surprising learning abilities. The study of brain evolution has made it possible to affirm that memory is established already in the first month of pregnancy, a memory that develops thanks to the stimulations that the child receives. Hearing voices, noises, sounds and music, the unborn child shows a remarkable capacity for discrimination. He appreciates the music of Mozart, Albinoni and Vivaldi and, whilst disapproving of rock music, does not hesitate to express his disappointment with strong kicks. However, the baby in utero is able to memorise the music that is heard during pregnancy and is able to recognise the tunes after birth. In moments of excitement, hearing these familiar tunes will calm him down as will the mother's voice. It is not only important to let the child listen to beautiful music, but it is essential to speak and sing to the child, because in this way a real knowledge is established in which the sound is the intermediary object that allows and facilitates the relationship, along with dialogue and empathy. Sound is a privileged vehicle of love between mother and child.

As you can see, it is mainly you mother, who can help the child to value all his innate gifts making him reach a series of stimulations, that will help him in his physical and mental evolution. *He will thus arrive at birth with an array of positive experiences.*

For example, stroking the baby bump and speaking softly to the child, will make him understand how much he is desired and loved. Furthermore, your caressing will stimulate his nervous system. The sweet melodies that you will make him listen to will not only give him the pleasure of hearing pleasant sounds, but also to promote the development of the brain. Moreover, the vibrations that come to his ear – which in the fifth month of pregnancy will have reached their final form – will contribute to the start for his love for music.

In essence, what is the primary need of a child in order to develop the potential to grow? *Not only must he feel loved, but also accepted, understood and listened to with the heart.* When the child feels listened to and you, mother, show it to him, the communication begins and from this, the relationship and attachment is commenced, thus giving way to a relationship that will continue in all subsequent phases, a relationship that will give the child that beneficial sense of security that will accompany him throughout his life. These are important imprints, which will help us live a socially balanced existence.

In your prayers and meditations, imagine him inside you sitting in the lotus position. It will be beneficial for your little one to feel included in your moments of spiritual elevation. All this will build up experiences in the child, that he will carry with him at birth and which will emerge in the following years in various forms, albeit all positive.

The participation of the father is extremely important for the development of the child. If the father will consciously follow all the phases of his child's formation, the mother-father-child triad will be created at the beginning, which will represent for the new being, the first experience of love. Whilst, for the couple it will represent the consolidation of their union. *Love and joy are two indispensable elements for the well-being of the child.* However, it must not fail to respect the work that is taking place inside him, if you consider how quickly and with how much wisdom the cells multiply in his little body, in order to reach the end of the ninth month with a complete and functioning structure. It is an extraordinary task which one never thinks about but is miraculous! So, not only love, but also a lot of respect should be given to the new creature, by everyone.

The most striking aspect of this fascinating period of human life is that mother and fetus, although united in the most intimate of physical relationships, are two distinct persons, each with their own project of life.

If you had to experience difficult moments – unfortunately, in the course of life you may experience moments of great pain, such as a grief or other feelings – it is good that you *explain to the child that he should not feel involved* because it happened, but that he should quietly continue to look after its growth, protected by the love of mum and dad who want nothing but its serenity. Explain to him that in life, things do not always go as we would like them to but that with goodwill, everything is smoothened. These words will help him shape a strong character, ready to understand situations and at the same time, eager for serenity.

You too, dad, can talk and play with your child. You can lightly tap the baby bump and receive, in answer, as many taps. This is a very amusing game that, if repeated, should be played in hours that are suitable for mom and dad because the child records the time of the game and, after the birth, punctually at that time the child will expect to play.

For you, woman who is experiencing a pregnancy, *this is the moment to become aware of your extraordinary potential that gives you the ability to manage such a big task:* to create and bring into your family, society and the whole world a healthy new person with a balanced body and mind, who is able to bring with him only those positive and constructive principles, which will improve the quality of life for future generations.

VIII

Gestation from the medical point of view

It is possible to divide the pregnancy into three trimesters, each characterized by a series of physical and emotional changes in the woman and by different sensations that pervade it.

1st Trimester *(from the last menstrual period to the end of the 13th week)*

This is certainly a very delicate period, in which many transformations take place, including the development of all the organs of the newborn. Important psycho-physical changes take place in it. There will be a modification of the hormonal structure, to allow the continuation of the pregnancy.

This period is certainly represented by an ambivalence: in fact, the impact and reaction with the diagnosis of pregnancy is complicated, whether it was wanted or not. In the future mother, mixed feelings arise: the conflict between the desire to continue to be herself and to become a mother.

It is absolutely normal to feel torn and poised between these two sensations. From a strictly physical point of view, the maternal body prepares itself to accept pregnancy. In the first few weeks, ailments such as nausea, a sense of turgidity and discomfort in the breasts, constipation and the increased need to urinate may appear.

2nd Trimester *(from the 14th to the 27th week)*

This period is characterised by the increase in the volume of the uterus: pregnancy becomes visible and becomes a "social event". The woman begins to perceive fetal movements (around the 18th-20th week).

The decision to accept pregnancy has been taken both physically and emotionally. This is the period of symbiosis with the child, of the encounter with its movements and its manifestations.

Nausea, vomiting and the frequent need to urinate usually disappear. However, varicosities and greater vaginal secretions may appear. The breasts increase in volume and stretch marks may appear as well as changes in skin color (face and mammary area).

3rd Trimester *(from the 28th to the 40th week)*

The fetus grows rapidly both in terms of size and functional capacities that develop. The woman begins to prepare herself for what will be the physical separation from her child and to think about birth. Towards the end of pregnancy, the newborn is also prepared for birth by settling in a cephalic position, that is upside down.

The future mother is more active and goes out from what was the state of absolute symbiosis with the newborn that had characterised the previous quarter. This is how the nesting instinct manifests itself: everything must be ready for the baby's arrival. This may also be a moment of ambivalence, in which the woman feels torn between the desire to see her child, to let him go, and to continue her pregnancy so as not to separate from him.

At the end of the trimester, the newborn moves downwards, getting sick in the mother's pelvis and the woman usually feels better, breathing and digesting more easily, even if the fatigue of nine months of pregnancy begins to be felt.

IX

Blessing ritual of an expectant mother

In my research on pregnancy and cultural stratifications that leads back to pregnancy, I came across this ritual that I find touching and that I would like to bring you back here. It is one of the rituals still used by the Indians of America. It is a party that takes place between women, to which only one man can be invited: the partner of the expectant mother.

It is necessary to gather: invitations, sage, flour of any cereal, a bowl, a jug of water, candles, gifts for the future mother (including her favourite foods), instruments for making music and a yarn of thread. The scent of sage is widespread to purify the space in which the ritual will take place. In the middle of the room there will be a carpet on which a small altar is created made up of candles, flowers, gifts, sacred objects and sweets. The guests sit in a circle, except for the mother who, in the middle of the carpet, lies on cushions next to the altarpiece, with her hair tied up and dressed in a loose and comfortable dress. Then the candles are lit and the purpose of the meeting is discussed. The mother will be celebrated with affectionate words, caresses, songs, gifts, as well as with her favourite food. One of the women will undo the mother's hair and brush it. Another woman will pour some water into a bowl containing the cereal flour and will knead the dough until a uniform cream is obtained, with which it will massage the hands and feet of the mother. After this, hands and feet are rinsed and dried with a soft cloth. All women participate in the cleansing and purification of the mother's body, manifesting tenderness and love. One woman can encourage her to take a dessert, others will present her with gifts. Meanwhile, some sing, others recite poems, share lived stories, laugh, cry, and others create moments of silence: all to celebrate the mother and give meaning to the sacred period she is experiencing. At one point, one of the women will take the yarn of thread and wrap the head of the thread around a mother's wrist. Then she will continue to wrap the thread around a wrist of all the women present, creating a real bond between them. When all women have their bracelet, the mother offers a prayer written on a piece of paper and which must be kept in a basket. Before concluding the ritual, the women separate themselves by cutting the thread that joined them, so that each one remains a bracelet to symbolize the loving bond that has firmly united them. Link that will manifest itself in a particularly explicit way during labour and delivery. The meeting ends with a prayer of thanksgiving and blessing.

X

The sound

Sound is a fascinating theme full of meaning. We are readdressed to the "verb" of St. John, the big bang, primordial symbols, the vibration of the divine breath that man has always conjugated with religious symbols. We speak of sacred sounds and sacred musical instruments.

Sound is a vibrational form of energy. The one who dealt with sound in relation to the theme of birth is certainly Alfred Tomatis, a French doctor, who passed away not many years ago. He writes:

> *Everything is sound [...]. The stars are the sounds, their planets and what is contained. Sound is the call of bodies, from the simplest to the most complex. The human being itself is sound, even if with time he has forgotten it.*

Starting from a strict subliminal vibrational-sound relationship between mother and fetus, Tomatis elaborates complex and fascinating theories, as well as important therapeutic methods based on sound.

We are interested in sound as a mother-fetus connection. At the beginning of gestation, sensory sensitivity increases, also in the direction of listening, in particular listening to oneself, which often tends to make even one's prenatal experience emerge.

Before the formation of the ear, the perception of sound by the fetus is left at the vibrational level, felt through the epidermis. Since the sound is energy, this is going to affect the brain of the fetus, constituting – warns Tomatis – a source of both psychological and physiological energy. One can therefore speak of sound stimulation of the nervous system.

The ear of the child is formed after 24 weeks and can therefore hear, even if not all frequencies; the amniotic liquid here is a filter. The sounds you get used to are repetitive or recurrent maternal sounds: heartbeat, blood flow, etc. but above all the voice of the mother, unique and inimitable.

This array of sounds, in addition to giving the child a sense of presence and a functional and physiological value, is also charged with very deep emotional values.

The child can also perceive the range of emotions with good precision. That's why it's so important to talk and sing to the child. The sound is the true vehicle of contact between mother and child!

Even the father can establish a sound link with the unborn child: the frequencies that are heard by the child are mainly intermediate ones, which correspond to the male voice.

If the father speaks 10-20 cm away from the womb, it is shown that the child feels and reacts, generally with kicks and somersaults, to position himself so that he can hear better!

Therefore, if the sounds generated by the mother, predominantly acute frequencies, vibrate at the nervous level, the paternal ones, more serious, vibrate at the bone and muscle level. While uterine sounds refer to an internal world, those paternal ones can represent a first door to the outside, a sort of preview of the world that is out there.

After birth, the child will recognise in that voice the profound bond that that voice subtended.

*There is a place where time
is not marked by the ticking of the clock,
but by the beating of the heart.*

Bianca Buchal

XI

Let us go to the music world…

If we keep in mind that the wise from the Far East have explained to us that "all creation is vibration", it is clear to us how important music is. Since we have learned that the child also hears the sounds coming from the outside and knows how to process and recognise them, the future mother cannot avoid introducing the world of sounds and music in her relationship with the child.

We do expect to raise so many Mozart's (by the way, what harmony did Mozart listen to before he was born, if he then played from three years onwards?), instead we aim to introduce the sound, the word, poetry, lullabies, nursery rhymes all told and sung by the mother.

Nursery rhymes and lullabies derive from a peasant culture, a group culture that handed down its traditions orally. It is not certain that the musical bases handed down to us are the original ones: many have been lost over time. Those who cannot sing can simply recite them, since even the word alone can have a musical effect. For an unborn child (or for a newborn) nothing has more value than friendly sounds that come from the mother's voice.

Many future Mothers ask me if the music should be divided

into two aspects: the prenatal one and the one related to the newborn. I always answer that this division does not exist. The newborn child will recognise sounds heard during pregnancy and will deduce consequent behaviours. How much crying can you avoid with some simple... "musical device" played at the right time!

Lullabies and nursery rhymes are back in vogue and are strongly recommended by psychologists. The unborn child or the newborn do not understand the logical meaning of the words, but rely on sensations, the sweetness of the mother's voice that tries to console them, a sound that always follows a loving act.

Personally, I recommend to expecting mothers to abandon themselves to long session of classical music or, in any case, quietly melodic. The selected musical pieces must always reflect one's own taste, preferably 18th century music, always in a higher tone (for example Mozart or Vivaldi).

Drumming, syncopated, strongly irregular rhythms certainly do not communicate calm, if anything they might alarm, cause disquietude and sometimes disharmony. So, expecting mothers, let's go slowly with disco evenings at 1000 watts or even just horror movies, with all the loud sound that they entail in the cinema! The child who was born who had to pass through moments of nervousness will have to be calmed. There is only one way to recite nursery rhymes and lullabies: the affective one. It is essential to transmit to the child all the love we feel for him.

XII

…and let's dress our life with colors

Every mother knows she can communicate with her child were already born. If she does so, it will create the most favourable conditions for the development of a balanced, healthy, energetic and beautiful qualities.

Also colors also have a precise role. Maybe not as intuitive as music, but it is still about vibrations. If we accept that chromotherapy has a role, then we will also admit that colors are very important in a period of our life in which we are more sensitive to what is happening around us.

If we want to find correspondence between music and colors, let's remember this musical correspondence…

- Do major: Red
- Re major: Orange
- Mi major: Yellow
- Fa major: Green
- Sol major: Blue
- La major: Indigo
- Si major: Purple

It is therefore important to dress up our outer world (and, as we will see later, also the inner world) of colors. In this regard, let us remember the meanings and values of each primary color...

- RED: is the color of life, of vitality, of dynamism, of will; strengthens the muscular system.
- ORANGE: is the color of health, of joy, of inner beauty, of transformation; affects the circulatory system, blood and heart.
- YELLOW: corresponds to intelligence, wisdom, reason; strengthens the central nervous system, the brain and the spinal cord.
- GREEN: is linked to growth, hope, abundance and birth; presides over the digestive system, the stomach and the intestine.
- BLUE: is the color of inner peace, of music, of truth and harmony; affects the lungs.
- INDIGO: develops nobility of thought, loyalty, stability, mastery; strengthens the bone system and the skin.
- PURPLE: inspires purity, develops imagination and intuition, exhorts altruism and compassion and is therefore linked to the spiritual values of human beings; acts on the hormonal system and strengthens the endocrine glands.

Even clothing will have to be rich in colors. Colors are vibrations, while black is complete absence of vibrations and, as such, absorbs everything, also impregnating itself with negative vibrations. Let us remember to furnish the house and dress ourselves with colors that bring joy, well-being, harmony. Let us now turn to the description of a simple but effective exercise to be carried out using the "magic" of colors ...

An easy and useful daily exercise

Gather seven sheets of the seven colors of the solar spectrum, in their purest scale. Whilst observing them, joy will be felt. Now, with your eyes closed, try to reproduce these same colors with your mind one by one. During this exercise, imagine the most beautiful qualities you want for your child. The mere fact of evoking them with thought is sufficient to ensure that the process that will act on the cellular memory of your child is introduced.

Now, for a preliminary relaxation, sit in a quiet place. Open your heart and let all the love you have for your baby flow and, if at the end of this work you listen to yourself, you will perceive what he will suggest to you.

Now inhale and exhale gently and slowly, like when you want to smell a flower. Then begin to breathe in alternate nostrils; then continue with both nostrils, imagining a beam of white light that wraps you completely. The white light will induce you to perform the following exercises in the best way.

Imagine now a red, luminous and shimmering flower. Inhale its color. Live intensely this beautiful red that goes to impregnate the cells of your child, bringing him energy and lots of love. Imagine him already born, while he runs and plays happily. He is a cheerful and confident child.

Now immerse yourself with your child in orange color. You see it rising from the bottom up to cover all the parts of your body. Inhaling, this color sends its vibrations to your child; list all the good qualities you would like to convey to them. Add the most beautiful expressions that flow from your heart to convey the pleasure of participating. Continue this exercise with commitment. Every day you can renew it by choosing another color and, therefore, other virtues. Let yourself be inspired by the moment and stimulate your imagination to create a fascinating scenario and bring to your imagination the most beautiful images.

For the color yellow, you can choose the sun, for the green the nature that awakens in the spring, for the blue a beautiful clear sky and for the purple a beam of pure and vibrant light that wraps you like a big spiral.

XIII

Centers for the accompanying towards pregnancy and childbirth

I see with great satisfaction that in recent years, even in Italy, Centers usually managed by midwives are flourishing. These Centers aim to accompany young expectant mothers along their path, according to new criteria and new methods that are also proposed in this book.

Perhaps the most original and probably also the first, is the *Heliotropium Centre* in Milan, that recently celebrated its twenty-five years of activity and that stems from the expertise, enthusiasm and inexhaustible vitality of Evelyne Disseau, a true Mother to expectant mothers. As in these cases, the Heliotropium is focused on the multiple experiences and skills of Evelyne, ranging from teaching yoga to astrology courses and much more.

The activities offered in these real Maternity Homes also take care of the mother's and child's body, offering numerous techniques to pamper yourself like a tender massage, or to treat oneself in an alternative way, for example with Bach flowers and essential oils.

Future mothers, but also fathers, participate enthusiastically and take courses to accompany pregnancy and childbirth.

Those who took part in the courses witness this experience with immense gratitude, remembering the interesting evenings spent with the group and recognising that they experienced a transformation from an uncertain, doubtful and frightened parent to a happy parent and aware of their role. These Centres also remain a very important reference point for the mother also after childbirth.

Blessed are the children who are born from parents that are well prepared on all levels, on everything that is useful to know in order to face pregnancy and the birth of their child, as well as in immediately creating a strong bond that lasts a lifetime!

*Fall asleep every night
with a serene thought:
lean your head on a pillow of clouds
and cover your body with a blanket of stars.
Reach unknown dimensions a day,
where sounds, colors and perfumes
become emotions.
Drop tension, anger, doubts and fear...
and rest, small still flame
in the heart of God.*

Sarasvati

XIV

Let's talk about nutrition

For the future health of the child, the appropriate diet to be observed during pregnancy will have to start long before conception.

First of all, it will be good to dispel the myth that "the pregnant woman has to eat for two". Instead, it will have to take care of two important things:

1. The quality of food, which must be free of preservatives, ideally biological and whole meal;
2. The amount of food, which will have to reach a total of about 2000/2500 calories daily, must never fall below 1600 calories.

This must be scrupulously observed, especially during the third trimester, in order not to slow down the growth of the child.

The diet may include: pasta, cereals, fish, vegetables, dairy products and fruit. If taken in reasonable quantities and in the right proportion, these foods will provide a balanced supply of proteins, vitamins, carbohydrates, lipids (fats) and mineral salts necessary to ensure the well-being of the mother and child.

It is advisable to eliminate fried food and elaborate sauces that are difficult to digest, without letting monotony take over, in order make meals a pleasant experience.

Weight gain during pregnancy

A woman in good health and with a weight that falls within the norm, should have gained 9-12 kg, distributed as follows:
- 1 kg per month for the first three months;
- 1-1.5 kg per month for the rest of the period.

If you are already overweight, you must scrupulously follow the doctor's advice.

There is a saying: "healthy body and mind"

We have seen what we must do to have a healthy body. What about the mind?

For the health of the mind it is good to eat slowly and chew for a long time, not only to facilitate the work of the stomach but also because the mouth, which is the first to receive food, is an important chemical laboratory. Moreover, the mouth does not process and only transform the material part of the food (starch in sugar, etc.), but also extracts some etheric particles that immediately feed the nervous system.

These are subtle substances, they give life to everything. Plants, earth, water, air, everything contains them, and it is thanks to these particles that everything lives and grows, even the stones. If the mother absorbs them, they will also reach the baby.

For those who have never deepened this field, be aware that the biological function takes place anyway, but it will be much more effective if accompanied by our awareness and our gratitude.

We must thank Nature for the solid and subtle substances contained in food, thank her for the variety of shapes, colors, flavours, perfumes ... always thank! It will also benefit the child, who will learn to love Nature.

*When women will once again become
the Priestesses of the cult of divine Love,
of Purity and of Grace,
men will learn the lesson
to become knights of the nobility again
and rediscover the qualities they have lost.
This will happen precisely thanks to women.*

Omraam Mikhaël Aïvanhov

XV

Smoking and alcohol during pregnancy

A healthy and serene child is born from a healthy and serene woman. No technological means can ever improve the process of physiological and spontaneous delivery, but only to disturb it.
Michel Odent

Smoking is always harmful for health but the greatest damage occurs when the woman smokes during pregnancy. Smoking causes adverse effects on the intrauterine environment and on the development of the fetus: abnormalities in insertion of the placenta, pre-term birth, decreased weight of the baby at birth, delay in intrauterine growth, behavioural abnormalities, etc.

These anomalies make it easy to understand the intensity of fetal suffering in having to undergo maternal smoking. Furthermore, cases of spontaneous abortion can occur. Even more concerning, is the fact that children born to women who continued to smoke during pregnancy have a high probability of being born underweight.

The consequences of the harmfulness of smoking during pregnancy are directly proportional to the daily dose of smoked cigarettes; remember also that if the mother smokes during pregnancy, the child will be more exposed to smoking addiction when he grows up.

For unrepentant pregnant women, a gradual reduction of the daily dose is advisable rather than a drastic cessation, in order to avoid unwanted psychological repercussions and unpleasant abstinence. There are various nicotine-based substitutes available in the pharmacy to help women quit smoking. However, be careful: passive smoking can also cause all the aforementioned risks.

The damage caused by alcohol is not lesser

It is now known that the consumption of alcoholic beverages during pregnancy is potentially very damaging to the child's growth. In order to not disturb its natural development, it is necessary to completely abolish the alcohol.

Four glasses a day and repeated states of intoxication are sufficient to disturb the course of gestation. Physical malformations and mental retardation may occur, which would cause severe discomfort to the child (difficulty in learning and socialising).

For the health of the mother and child, abstinence from alcohol is therefore strongly recommended.

It should be kept in mind that the inflow of oxygen is essential to guarantee your child a normal and quiet growth!

XVI

The mother's stress on the quality of fetal life

Stress, in substance, is the inability of the organism to adapt itself to changed conditions of one's inner or outer environment. It is distinguished in acute, sub-acute and chronic stress, obviously according to the duration of the condition of inadequacy.

Prolonged stress leads to negative consequences on pregnancy, just as chronic anxiety leads to an increase in the rate of pregnancy arrest, delayed fetal growth and an alteration of the placental morphology. Recent American and French studies demonstrate this very clearly. In particular, a study conducted by Rosalind Wright of Harvard Medical School in Boston, presented in May 2008 at the American Thoracic Society's international congress in Toronto, shows that the mother's stress could predispose her baby to allergies and asthma.

Acute stresses in the first three months of gestation can cause various effects: for example, not infrequently, strong differences in dermatology (fingertips) between right and left hands arise.

In the following three months, characterised by a strong development of neurons in the cerebral cortex, acute stress can determine sensitive psychological and behavioural effects.

A study of a few decades ago showed that subjects whose father had died before birth often were the protagonists of asocial acts and presented psychiatric disorders with frequencies much higher than the control group.

It should be stressed, however, that these studies are very difficult: it is not easy to classify the type of stress of the mother. In fact, behaviour often tends to "mask" anxious states and we do not underestimate the protective role of the mother! Just think of all those pregnancies that occurred under dramatic conditions in World War II, which also gave birth to perfectly normal children.

We must not underestimate the excessive fatigue of the mother, which implies a greater consumption of oxygen on her part, to the detriment of the child who, instead of growing harmoniously needs regular oxygenation.

It is however evident that pregnancy requires a condition of maximum serenity. Here too, mind you, first of all naturalness. In addition, I like to think about the topic of stress by using positive rather than negative images. The constant accounting of stress on the part of the pregnant woman would in turn be anxious and so, on the understanding that the maternal-fetal relationship of negative emotions is clarified, the solution is to succeed in giving life to a constant, spontaneous positive current of joy (which cannot certainly be originated on command) and of Love (which, however, is free to flow to the unborn child at any moment he allows it).

In short: joy and love are the best antidotes to the negative effects of stress!

XVII

Some advice for a conscious, positive and happy pregnancy

Here is a list of simple and effective tips and activities. By controlling your thoughts, your feelings and taking on a harmonious behaviour, you will favour in your child:

1. The building of his health and will

- Choose healthy foods;
- Prepare your meals with joy;
- Avoid alcohol and tobacco so as not to poison your own child and not plant in him the predisposition to smoke;
- Breathe for two: slow and deep breathing gives life and harmony to energy;

2. The taste of beauty and its ability to love

- In communicating with your child, send him a lot of Love;
- Calm him down if you feel worried or angry;
- Talk to him as if he were already born;
- Sing for him to make it vibrate at the sound of your voice;
- Admire the beauties of nature and works of art;

- Be spontaneous and establish a link with him according your character and culture;
- Look for everything that harmonises and gives you pleasure, remaining in constant contact with him;
- Avoid anything that could upset you and your child (negative conversations, sad readings, depressing feelings, violent and destructive music and images, fears and uncertainties ...);

3. A creative and universal intelligence

- Face the difficulties of life with the certainty of overcoming them: the character and the will of your child will be strengthened;
- Concentrate your thinking and your imagination on the most beautiful human qualities: your child will bring with him the seed for a better world!

VIII

The massage

Hippocrates, "father" of western medicine, as early as the 5th century BC, wrote that: *"The doctor must know how to do various things, but he certainly must know how to massage"*, and that *"massaging is a method for health and longevity"*.

The massage is present in every culture and in every age – from the Chinese to Ayurvedic Indians to Middle Eastern cultures – with the common idea that health and well-being are the result of an energetic and functional rebalancing.

On the physiological side, the massage revitalizes, tones the muscles, stimulates fluid exchange, oxygenation, lymphatic and blood circulation, it sedates the nervous system, lowers the pressure, normalises breathing. Those who receive the massage produce endorphins, establish an empathic relationship with those who perform it, activate the right cerebral hemisphere that presides over perception.

All this opens the way to a clearer feeling and it is a bridge towards ourselves. A quiet mind and accentuated feelings lead us into dimensions that are often difficult to contact in the everyday hectic life. How does the massage enter our birth path? In two ways. Firstly, the massaging of an expecting mother which serves to accompany the woman, to relaxation and to the creation of a channel of communication between mother and child on a physical, energetical and emotional level. The ideal frequency would be at least once a week. The best months are from the third to the sixth. Thereafter, the massage will focus on the lumbar area and on the belly.

Ideally the massage should be performed by the partner which would complete the parent-child triangle. In any case, whoever does it must be willing to properly learn the technique and to do it with due caution. However, if it is considered useful to add techniques such as acupressure, plantar reflexology and "light massage" a specialisation is needed. These techniques can even be used to intervene on the child's position or on structural and functional problems of the woman in the last months of pregnancy.

Subsequently, there is the role of the massage practiced on the newborn, whose specific technique must be learned. After the separation from the mother, that is often traumatic and prolonged, the child will feel the need to restore a skin contact, a deep, warm, enveloping relationship, where the hands send the skin a loving message and a warm embrace. A non-verbal language to which, once again, the father can participate.

In addition to the bath, a nice daily massage will help the baby grow stronger and healthier, helping him to eat better, sleep better and avoid those small illnesses that are so frequent in the first months of life. Over time, the contact of the skins, with all the meanings it conveys, will gradually become more intense and conscious. Ideally, it would last until the 18th-24th month.

From joy flows creation,
from joy it is sustained,
towards joy it proceeds
and to joy it returns.

Mundaka Upanishad

XIX

A child speaks to his parents from the womb

A child speaking from the womb:

I am happy that you gave me the opportunity to communicate with the world, because I have so many things to say, also in the name of all children: those close to birth but also those that will be conceived in the future.

First of all, I would like to thank my mother who, with a lot of sweetness does not only provide me with the nourishment needed for the construction of my body but also demonstrates tenderness in various forms. I feel all these things, I feel that she already loves me very much and looks forward to the day when she can hold me in her arms. I too cannot wait for that moment to come, to know her face, her smell and her warmth! We must wait patiently. Meanwhile, I like to hear her voice, especially when she speaks to me. Even if it does so only with thought, I perceive it, because in this long nine-month period we are a single being, even if at the same time, we are two distinct persons, each with its own destiny and with its own life plan.

As I feel her thoughts, I also understand her feelings and I rejoice when I feel she is serene and calm. If she's quiet, I too can be quiet; and, when I'm quiet, I can take better care of building the cells that will form all the different parts of my little body. It's a big job, but my mother ensures that all the purest and most necessary substances come to me. I am very grateful to you because everything that you send me is full of love. Her thoughts and feelings, everything is soaked

with love and this is how I receive the necessary elements to form my mind. This cooperation is beautiful.
Thanks Mom!

I love it when she sings for me! I have heard that hearing good music is good for me and helps me grow. Mum knows many beautiful songs. There are some sweet lullabies, and I'm sure she'll sing them to me later, when I'm in my crib. Hearing the songs that I already know, in moments of agitation will certainly calm me down because I will understand that birth was only a transition from the first phase to the next.
Maybe that's why my ears are already able to hear, to memorise everything from now and to better recognise and appreciate it later. In fact, I know all the sounds of my "outside" house: the telephone, the vacuum... but what I like most is the voice of my mother, not only when she speaks to me but especially when she sings. Five months have passed and I am already able to participate in everything that happens in the surrounding world. I do not only recognise the voice of my mother, but also the more serious one of my father. It is so nice when I am caressed! In fact, he caresses my mother's belly, but I feel it's him. It's a special touch that makes me joyful all the time. When we play "soccer", I enjoy it very much! Mum and dad have fun too because they feel my presence and I am happier than they are because I feel I am awaited and loved. In fact, for us children, Love is a fundamental nourishment.
I am sorry for all the children who in the past have not been able to experience these moments of joy. Once, everyone believed that before birth, we were very small insensitive beings, unable to perceive anything, not even physical pain. They said that only at birth would we become a person, they used to consider us only a mass of cells. Only our mothers

took us into their hearts. Unfortunately, sometimes, not even them (but I do not want to talk about this because it's too painful!).
Now everything is different and we owe it to the many researchers and scholars who have been probing the world in mummy's belly for so many years. They can do it because now they have appliances, but we do not like them at all, as they are terribly noisy. It is true, however, that now mum and dad can observe us on a window and in them, this possibility triggers a strong emotion, since they are faced with a reality that previously, was only a dream.
They can see us suck our thumbs or while we pee, they see us as we move and very often, they even manage to figure out if we are a boy or a girl. Usually it's the father who would like to know, while the mother says it's not important for her, as long as the child is healthy.
Meanwhile, the doctors look at us, they check us, measure us and judge if everything is going well. For us, however, it is not so pleasant – I have heard that we will all be a generation of young helicopter lovers, because the apparatus that scrutinises us makes the same noise.
Sometimes they access the bag that holds us with a very long needle to extract some liquid, and that's scary. I know that some children manage to push the needle away due to fear of being harmed. These are all strange things but they say they are important. However, we must be grateful to all researchers because they give us the attention we deserve, making sure that even when we are born we are taken into account and treated in the correct way because we also have needs, not just newborns. One thing that I really like is when mum and dad go for a walk in the middle of nature. On those occasions, I can feel the positive effect of something they call "oxygen". They say it is very important for the

formation of our brain. They say that when the brain is well developed, it also benefits all the other organs. In fact, I feel that it is just like that. I really hope that mum and dad often go for a walk in the countryside, not only for me, but also because it is very beneficial for them. They spend most of their time at work, so these beautiful walks in nature are moments of intimacy that include me as well – because their conversations are always aimed at the future, with their child. These experiences help consolidate what they call bonding, the mom-dad-child "bond", which will keep us close and united even afterwards. This union gives me a lot of peace and security because I feel that I will always find in them great and sincere friends.

I'm glad to have said all these things. There would be many more things to add, but I will say them some other time. Oh, no, I still have two things to say: one is that when I will be born, I would like my dad to be with us, to assist and be close by and I am certain that mum would want it too. The second is that, immediately after my birth, I will need to stay with my mother. The transition from fetus to child is a very delicate moment and close to my mother, I will feel more protected and safe. As soon as I am born, it is important that I remain close to my mother as I want to meet her gaze and receive her kisses and caresses. We must stay together to give birth to all those feelings we have dreamed of, in the previous months. What a great joy it will be to be held in her arms!

Even dad's will be very important. I would like him to cut the umbilical cord and separate me from my mother to start our family. It would be nice if it was dad who gave me the first bath. We children are very sensitive to these loving attentions, they help us create a joyful beginning to our existence in the world. Everyone will ask themselves: but how can he understand, how can he distinguish words, how can he hear what they say to him? In fact, it is not the meaning of the words that come to me but that flow of profound feelings that overcomes all the barriers, which does not require phrases or concepts but which goes directly to my little heart, always very sensitive and open to every sincere and loving feeling.

This is how I am so confident in my life in the world and I feel that I will be a positive creature, firstly thanks to my mother but also to my father and to all those that awaited me with so much love.

I would also like to add that in the "Charter of Children's Rights", the rights of unborn children should also be contemplated. In fact, we would like to assert our right to be born in a family that has conceived us because it really desired us, that loves us already although it does not know us personally and that it can give us everything we need to lead a healthy life, full of interests that are able to trigger our physical and mental growth.

We do not have many expectations: we only need to be loved, because for us Love is food and if we receive a lot of love today, when we grow up we will give it back a hundredfold, for the good of all.

With so much gratitude

A prenatal child

*I did not notice the moment when
I crossed the threshold of this life for the first time.
What was the power that hatched me
in this vast mystery, like a flower blossoms
in a forest at midnight?
When I looked at the light in the morning
I immediately felt that
I was not a stranger in this world,
that the inscrutable without name
and without form
had taken me in his arms
in the form of my mother.
Thus, in death, the same stranger
will appear to me as always known.
And, because I love this life,
I know that I will also love death.*

Rabindranath Tagore

XX

The choice of the clinic

Giving birth is one of the normal functions of the woman's body, a function for which all women are perfectly prepared and adequate, thanks to the natural selection of species, perfected over millions of years!

Nowadays, the future mother often feels worried or unprepared at birth and therefore, many times, chooses the hospital focusing on the time of delivery; just as often she relies on the gynaecologist to choose the place of delivery, which in the vast majority of cases will be the hospital. The mothers who choose to give birth at home, in fact, are very rare in Italy. There is however an aspect in this choice that is often underestimated: breastfeeding.

In fact, choosing where you will give birth will be fundamental to making breastfeeding start "on the right foot". Pregnancy, childbirth and breastfeeding are not three separate moments that are only coincidentally close due to chronological reasons. They are an inseparable biological continuum and therefore, as such, each moment affects and influences the other.

At the moment of birth, the most ancient part of our brain is activated, the part devoted to the fundamental and ancestral functions, that are necessary for the survival of the species. A biochemical cascade of hormones is activated, which all perfectly with each other, to allow us to make our body and that of the child, work in the best way.

However, when birth does not happen as Nature forecasted, this mechanism can get stuck and therefore the new mother and the newborn may find themselves in trouble and instinct is no longer enough to make things go as they should. The hospital routine often creates various obstacles to this natural process that also interferes with breastfeeding.

A Swedish research conducted in 1990 (*The delivery self-attachment*, Righard & Alade, 1990) demonstrated that children born without hospitalisation and without separation from their mother were all perfectly able to "climb" on their mother's belly and to find the nipple, after which they all perfectly attached to the breast within a maximum of about 90 minutes from birth. Instead, when there had been a hospitalisation and/or mother-child separation, the percentage of capable children decreased drastically, many seemed confused and did not know what to do, others were frustrated and had to be helped because they were no longer able to find the mother's breast by themselves.

It has also been demonstrated, with a considerable amount of scientific evidence, that one of the crucial aspects for successful breastfeeding is the first breastfeed, implying that mother and child are not separated after birth and that the child can attach himself.

Another aspect of central importance is the possibility that even after giving birth, mother and child are not separated, so that the newborn has free access to the breast every time and for how long he wants. The mother will then sharpen her ability to understand the signs of hunger of her child. To this end, the so-called *Rooming-in* is essential, meaning that the child is in the room with the mother 24 hours a day.

It is often explained to the mother that it is healthier for her, for the child to be taken away right after birth, to make her rest, etc. In reality this can be very counterproductive. Scientific research has shown that mothers who sleep with their children, might certainly sleep less but definitely have a better quality of sleep and feel more rested, in comparison to sleeping far from their children.

For mothers who are convinced that they need to give birth according to new methods, the issue of how to overcome the rigid system of protocols arises. Protocols are comfortable as they refer to a routine and, moreover, represent a strong legal protection in the event of accidents and objections towards doctors, midwives and operators in general. In Italy, there are now numerous cases of mothers who, thanks to their obstinacy and determination, have succeeded in working with protocols, midwives and doctors to achieve their wishes. I encourage you to read the insights included in the next chapters: "Welcoming the Child at Birth" and "The Breastfeeding".

*What we understand when we look at things
is only part of things.
What gushes from our spirit
when it places itself in front of things
is the other part of it.
Things that speak to us from the outside
and things that speak
from our inner world
are the same,
but only when we join
the language of the external world
with our inner world
will we have full Reality.*

Rudolph Steiner

XXI

My childbirth: a magical event

Let us now read Mariasole's beautiful experience:

Emotions immediately arise to my throat and fill my eyes with warm tears, when I relive in my mind the highlights of Serena's birth: my second-born, born May 20th, 2002, at 00.52. Born in the sense that she saw the light, but even before conceiving her I felt her close and spoke to her. The nine months with her in the belly were a real joyous party: I felt very well both inside and outside. Jacopo, my first child, is 22 months old and not a day passed without us talking about Serena. My husband, Jacopo, and I awaited with happiness for the great birth event: there was too much desire to see our Serena! We all lived and experienced labour, childbirth and the entire pregnancy together. Every emotion, every game, every shopping at the supermarket, every ultrasound, every laugh, every speech: all together with Jacopo. All together we left for Florence, where there is a Maternity House. They welcomed us like family and our Jacopo was with me and my husband all the time – only one day – because we chose to be dismissed early in order to head home as soon as possible. On Sunday, May 21st, we spent it between contractions, walking in the garden of the hospital and feeling free in the Labour Hall with yellow walls. I breathed deeply and Serena slowly adapted to the big event. Jacopo imitated me and breathed deeply too and sometimes hugged me tightly! Meanwhile, the desire to meet Serena's gaze increased, but she took time and chose the night to get out of her sweet refuge in which she had been cradled and massaged for nine months. After dinner – I drank only water, lemon juice and honey to give the best of my energy to Serena – we played together and at 10pm Jacopo fell asleep. Francesca and I, the midwife, retreated near the beautiful pool for the birth and here, our last journey towards this fantastic experience began. My husband watched over Jacopo and occasionally came to see me: it was amazing when he found me already in the water at 37 degrees. I was very well and I was ready to face the last part of labour and delivery. Everything was done in a natural way. No oxytocin, no episiotomy, no elastic bands on the belly. We only monitored Serena's little heart from time to time, but it was all regular. The water had been salted and I felt light, open, free to float and happy. I never stopped being happy. I was happy because Jacopo was with us and, if he woke up and looked for me, he could see me right away. I was happy because I could have soon embraced Serena. Towards midnight, I told my Midwife about my birth. I was born dead, and talking about it helped me even more to free myself from this memory. I really want to live, thanks to the experience I had during birth! Jacopo had awakened after midnight, just as Serena was being born. What a joy to be an instrument of Life! So, while I was the first to greet sweet Serena with my hands and laid her on my chest in the water, my husband came along with Jacopo in his arms and we all looked at each other with great euphoria! Serena did not cry, she looked satisfied, the lights were soft and I spoke to her softly, saying, "You're beautiful, you'll have a wonderful life!" I stayed in the water with Serena for another forty minutes, after which the father cut the umbilical cord. We then settled on a round bed. Jacopo, Serena and I hugged each other for an hour. Daddy recorded us while Jacopo was kissing Serena. The first bath, or rather the second, I did with my hands: it was wonderful. The next morning, at 9:00 we were released and at 10:00 we were already at home. I placed Serena's placenta under a beautiful red flower in the garden as that placenta was her home for nine months.

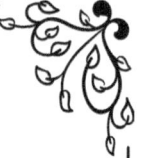

*Water has always been
the symbol of the mother at all times.
Life started from the ocean.
In the amniotic fluid
we recapture the history of our life.*

Michel Odent

XXII

Ode to birth

This chapter is also dedicated to a guided meditation taken from the book *Welcoming the Soul of a Child*, written by Jill Hopkins:

> You will need: incense sticks, a candle, rose or lavender scented water, material to draw or paint, sacred objects – anything that has special significance – and pillows.
> In the place that you have chosen – if you give birth at home, in the room where your child will be born – sit comfortably. Spread the scent of incense in the environment and pour some rose or lavender water into a basin. Light the candle and focus on your breath. Mentally, or loudly, pronounce the purpose of the ritual:
>
> MEDITATION ON THE DATE OF BIRTH.

> The day of your child's birth is approaching. You are counting down. The following meditation will help you generate a suitable atmosphere to welcome your child well; to help you, mother, to be more relaxed and also you, partner, to participate in this unforgettable event.
> Lie down and stay in this position for as long as you like. Meanwhile, simply, breathe. Breathe slowly and deeply. Imagine that all the worries, all the tensions, all the fears connected with the birth, basically all your thoughts, vanish with every exhalation. Imagine that air, rather than entering you through your nose or mouth, penetrates through the entire surface of your body so that the whole surface of

your skin becomes your respiratory organ. Take time to learn how to breathe this way. Without forcing yourself, let your breath become even deeper.

While breathing with your whole body, be aware of the air you breathe in. Imagine that air penetrating into every cell of your body: where you feel tired, it regenerates you; where you feel tension, it relaxes you; where you feel the emptiness, it fills you with light and life.

At this point, just imagine the environment in which you would like to welcome your child. Where would you like your child to be born?

- On the shore of the ocean, between the shells and the spray of water that smells of saltiness;
- At night, wrapped in silence, under a starry sky;
- At the foot of a giant oak, sensing the strength of his age;
- In spring, in a meadow full of flowers of all colors;
- In a field of ripe wheat, experimenting it's fertility;
- On the bare earth, under a rainbow;
- Under a gentle drizzle;
- Next to a waterfall;
- In the mountains, caressed by a breath of sparkling air;
- At sunrise or sunset...

These are just a few examples. It's up to you to imagine the environment you prefer.

Whatever the place you choose, view it with the utmost clarity. Imagine being there. Breathe and feel the scents, the tactile sensations, hear the sounds and seize the bright colors. As you repeat this exercise, the images will become more vivid and clearer. Do not feel discouraged if the first time is difficult. By continuing to view the same image, you will make it ever more real. Whatever the environment in which you would like to find yourself, in the vast space of the mind and thanks to the resources of your imagination, little by little you will create a living reality in your inner world and in the inner world of your child.

Imagine holding your child in your arms, just born. Communicate with him with words and songs, or through your skin.

Talk to him about the world in which he will soon be born and surround him with loving tenderness.

When you open your eyes, slowly return to your normal state and try to draw or paint the place you've chosen to give birth to your child. Remember that perfection and style are of no importance. Simply express it in the way that you feel to be the easiest. Complete the ritual with expressions of gratitude and display your design where you can always see it.

*A child who is born is not born by chance.
If you ask me why your son was born,
he will answer: "So that you know
what you have in your mind".
This is how men and women learn
to know each other: through their children.*

Omraam Mikhaël Aïvanhov

XXIII

The pain of labour

Women! We possess all the knowledge and power necessary to give birth to our children. Let's do it with our resources and live it as an experience of health, growth and transformation.

These wise words can be read on one of the many Internet sites that deal with birth. Generally, we speak of pain to describe a sensation that is very complex to define: sensation which, on the contrary, possesses a great quantity of nuances, even of pleasure.

Medicine, with the desire to abolish pain, creates an unbeatable distance between the woman that is in the process of giving birth and her body. By offering the application of various analgesic techniques, medicine denies the woman the opportunity to know and express herself.

In the same way as all the physiological functions of the human body, the woman should be aware that her body is naturally also predisposed to the function of giving birth.

If fears and tensions have been created around this function, there obviously are reasons, reasons that must be understood and possibly overcome.

Preparation to childbirth courses have as their main purpose that of "informing" the woman, helping her to obtain an acceptable response to the pain she will have to face when her baby is born. In fact, the more you give pain a clear explanation and a convincing meaning, the more you raise the threshold of tolerability.

Giving meaning to the pain of labour, means to understand the reasons that encourage the woman to accept to live it. This will represent a profound physical and mental experience for the woman that, however, has nothing pathological. Moreover, it is an evil that, when it is finished, is completely forgotten.

It is certain that when a woman faces childbirth, in all its phases, with a natural approach, she is satisfied, and this feeling will be reflected on many aspects of *"post-partum"* and beyond, not only on herself, but also on the born child.

It is important, however, that the delivery room is filled with a serene and peaceful atmosphere, to allow the woman to experience, possibly with her partner, this unforgettable "moment" in all tranquillity and concentration, avoiding distractions and interruptions that would prolong the duration of the process.

XXIV

Caesarean section

This is an ancient surgery. Many historians attribute the term "caesarean section" to the birth of Julius Caesar who, according to the myth, was born in this way. However, it also is true that an ancient Roman law under the king Numa Pompilius, named *lex cesarea*, prescribed the abdominal extraction of the fetus from all pregnant women who died at the end of pregnancy.

The first caesarean section documented on a living woman, but who died a few days later, dates back to 1610; it is only in 1794 that the first woman survives the surgery. Still in 1865 the maternal mortality was equal to 85% of the surgeries! The lack of antibiotics, the lack of understanding of the need to sew the uterine wound, the technique of incision that, for a long time, occurred longitudinally on the most vascularised part of the uterus and the lack of a suitable anaesthesia caused the maternal and fetal mortality level to be very high for long period of time.

Benefits, but also risks

Information is important. Undoubtedly, the caesarean section has changed the history of child birth, contributing significantly to drastically reducing maternal mortality and maternal diseases resulting from childbirth. At the same time, its benefits on the fetal-neonatal front were extremely important.

In recent decades, the caesarean section technique has been perfected so much so that it can now be considered of very safe, but certainly never free from risks, particularly for the mother: anaesthesia, infections, haemorrhages, injuries to the ureters and bladder, cardio-pulmonary and thromboembolic complications, even if very limited.

It would advisable, if every pregnant woman were already informed during childbirth preparation courses, on the operative procedures of a caesarean section. In the event of an absolute emergency, being informed will help to deal with the surgery with greater awareness and less fear.

Natural childbirth is gratifying

Spontaneous birth is undoubtedly a very gratifying experience for the woman but, when the situation is difficult and risky, the caesarean section is very welcome.

There are women who consider caesarean sections a liberation from the suffering of labour. In this case, it is a decision that they make because they probably do not know that with the caesarean section, they miss the extraordinary values of the most important moment in the life of every woman: the birth of their child. In fact, in the final phase of childbirth, both the mother and the child secrete a hormone (*oxytocin*) which is called the "love hormone". When the child, with the umbilical cord still intact, is placed in the arms of the mother, where their eyes will meet for the first time – a magical moment – the oxytocin will facilitate mutual recognition, mutual attachment and mutual belonging, feelings that will last a lifetime.

For other women – and precisely when there is a high risk for both mother and child – a caesarean section is considered a salvation. For others, it is a failure because, without adequate information, they will later realise that they have renounced to something irretrievable, thus creating a void that will manifest itself in various forms during the life of both the mother and the child.

Or they will realise that, in exchange for a few hours of painful labour, they will then find themselves having to endure other, perhaps even more serious, long-lasting problems.

Reducing caesarean sections

The press provides endless statistics that provide information on the increasing growth of caesarean sections, worldwide. If we want to reduce this wave, which has even become slightly fashionable, I believe it is urgent to provide detailed information on a large scale, to enable all concerned women to truly learn what the real difference between caesarean sections and natural delivery is, in order for them to make an informed decision.

However, it is assumed that following Nature is the wisest choice and it must be remembered that the woman's body possesses all the necessary characteristics to endure childbirth.

Doctors must remember that pregnancy is not a disease and that childbirth is not a surgical operation and it must be "humanised" in order to respect women and children. The same applies to epidural anaesthesia.

Here too, I invite you to read a few insights in the following chapters: "Welcoming the Child at Birth" and "The Wound that Medicine does not recognise".

XXV

Childbirth in water

Among the various options offered to the mother, who is preparing for childbirth, there is "birth in water" – made famous by studies conducted after 1980, but still not widespread.

Water is an element that attracts, contains, supports, caresses, massages and envelops. With its color, movement, rhythm and noise it is able to evoke pleasing, relaxing and attractive images and sensations.

Water is a symbol of femininity and is a source of life. Hot water facilitates a pleasant regression towards a state of sensorial well-being and invites one to let go. Water facilitates the perception of one's own body, with its own feelings and processes. Water allows one to let go and savour a deep and gratifying state of relaxation.

During labour, water is able to change the feelings in body, the perception of pain, time and space, providing relief, lightness and a subtle massage. For women, water facilitates relaxation, isolation from external stimuli, easier contact with one's most intimate parts and with one's instinctual dimension. Water, with its own instinctual symbology, reconnects the woman to that primitive wisdom that advises her what she must do and how she must do it. Even the unborn child receives multiple benefits, one of which is the welcoming, which takes place in a more relaxed atmosphere. For the child, the transition from a liquid environment inside the mother to an external aquatic one is certainly more delicate and less traumatic. Finally, water protects the baby's body from psychological effects, triggered by a sudden exposure to gravity. It appears that babies born with water birth have developed intuitive skills as well as a higher level of sensitivity.

Water can take on a deeper meaning if the birth event is associated with a sacred dimension of psychological and spiritual transformation.

Here are the benefits of childbirth in water:

1. Immersion in water lightens: the immersed body weighs 1/6 of when it is on the ground, so it relieves the weight of the baby bump, lightening the kidneys, the lumbar area and other internal organs;
2. Movements become easier, in the water we are more agile, we move more easily, less painfully (and movement during labour is essential...);
3. The pelvis is more mobile in its joints and the descent of the baby in the birth canal is more simple and natural;
4. Hot water relaxes all the muscles. Tensions disappear, the body breathes more deeply and regularly, it oxygenates more deeply and the mind is able to relax more easily, encouraging the recovery of energy. Muscles and

tissues of the uterine cervix, which expand faster and the structures that shape the birth canal, also become relaxed, making the child's transit easier and less painful;
5. Water softens the tissues: therefore, at the time of delivery, the risk of tearing decreases;
6. For the child, being born in water implies phasing more gradually from intrauterine to extra uterine life;

On the other hand, there may also be some disadvantages. As the well-known French gynaecologist Michel Odent suggests, there is no need to plan the water birth "with stiffness". The method and the opportunity must be discussed from time to time with the assisting medical team. Odent also advises spend only the labour phase, in water.

Welcome among us You are born

and from Light you come down into my arms,
hot circle of Love,
sweetness that cradles you on pink waves.
Every tension melts in an embrace
and your little heart looks for the rhythm
of the bigger heart that has protected him
for so many months in the long wait.
Welcome among us,
ancient spirit dressed in a new candid dress.
Welcome among us,
little life, thirsty of Light and Love.

Joy

XXVI

Labour and childbirth

Labour

The long months of pregnancy are about to come to an end. The birth is imminent and in the final days of waiting there is a feeling of "rehearsals". The child is preparing to enter the world and it is he who, working with his mother, gives way to labour.

Three to four weeks before birth – the period is variable – the child sits upside down, approaching the neck of the uterus. Now, it moves less due to the reduced available space; however, a minimum amount of movement is necessary to signal that, while waiting for the "big event", the little one is well.

Meanwhile, in the mother's organism the secretion of a series of hormones occurs, a secretion to which the child also contributes. The hormones in question are those that will trigger the labour. The main hormone is oxytocin, produced by both women and children. It is proof that in this important phase there is, between the two, a perfect and wonderful cooperation.

For the little one, it is not only a matter of preparing for the enormous physical effort that is necessary to overcome the complex transit through the birth canal, but also the encounter with a totally new environment.

For the woman, these hormones give way to labour, with light and distanced pains, pains that gradually intensify in strength and frequency. This phase can have a variable duration but the woman, becoming courageous, knows that she has to face and endure it patiently. However, every woman follows her own rhythm and the assistants must respect her...

Depending on the interpretation that is given to pain, it can be said that the more a meaning is attributed to it, the higher the threshold of tolerability is raised. Providing a meaning to the pain of childbirth, signifies having good reasons of allowing this profound mental and physical experience to occur.

The medical system, with its rule of "avoiding pain", tends to create a distance between the woman and her body, between the woman and her sensations, preventing her from feeling, knowing and expressing herself. The woman should know that her body is perfectly intended to perform the function of giving birth, as it is for any other function: to breathe, to digest...

The basic purpose of birth preparation courses – not just important but necessary! – is to lead the woman to give an answer to her suffering, working towards eradicating fear and tension. Providing a positive interpretation to the pain of childbirth, means transforming it and actively experiencing it as an opportunity for growth and not as a condemnation.

Childbirth

Let us now read the beautiful words of the French gynaecologist and midwife Frédérick Leboyer (taken from the book *Birth Without Violence*):

> Here, everything is ready: dimmed lights, music in the background, recollection... the child can arrive... Here it is! First the head comes out and then the arms... The baby is born! What more suitable place to lay it if not the mother's womb? The womb of the woman has the shape, the fit that is suitable for the child. Convex before, concave later; it seems to be waiting, like a nest. Its warmth, its elasticity, the fact that it rises and falls according to the rhythm of breathing, the sweetness, the warmth of the skin, all make it the perfect place where to lay down the newborn baby.

We can now move on to the next chapter, "Welcoming the Child at Birth"...

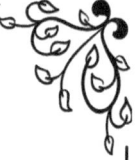

*Observe Nature and take care
of your little seed as she does.
Give her the strong energy
of the Earth with healthy food.
Give her the energy of water
with its purest emotions.
Caress her with the energy of the Air.
Give her elevated thoughts.
Illuminate her with the energy of the Sun
by offering her your Love.
The Plant-Man that will be born
will be strong and well rooted to the ground,
but with arms extended towards the Sky,
towards Freedom.*

Sarasvati

XXVII

"Obstetrician" and Midwife

In Italy, the future mother almost always and immediately turns to the gynaecologist. In reality, also with reference to Law n. 740, issued in 1994, the midwife is the ideal figure and role to monitor the woman from adolescence up until the senile age, facing the natural, physiological events related to the phases of the woman's life cycle: intrauterine life, birth, puberty, the adolescence, pregnancy, childbirth, fertile age and menopause.

In short, today the midwife has a set of technical, scientific and cultural skills that allows her to face the health problems of women, couples and families.

However, we said that in Italy, a pregnant woman automatically turns to the gynaecologist; the future mother is not aware of the fact that even a midwife is able to follow her in a physiological pregnancy. Midwives can follow future mothers in their pregnancy as freelancers or consultants. However, most women are unaware of this.

In recent years, many private "Accompaniment Centres' managed by midwives have been created but many women are still unaware of this option and often underestimate them by becoming afraid of the costs that may be incurred and failing to understand how important a targeted path in a cosy and quiet place and a respected birth is, for the future of their children.

In some regions of Italy there are basic national contributions for those who chose to give birth to their child at home or in a maternity centre and in some hospitals, birth centres have been opened, only managed by midwives, for those who want to experience a less medicalised birth.

The comparison with the English situation is interesting. In this case too, the United Kingdom provides us with an example of simplicity and efficiency. A pregnant woman in the United Kingdom is referred to the general practitioner, who will direct her to a community midwife, such as a local midwife. In cases where the pregnancy is not physiological, the midwife, assisted by the gynaecologist, will take care of the relationship with the woman and will remain present as a reference figure. If it proves necessary, she will refer her to a medical specialist.

The fact of being present locally is an advantage: the territorial proximity, which leads to more frequent and close relationships as well as the overall tranquillity and serenity of knowing that you are close to a professional, during the entire pregnancy.

It is essential for the British healthcare system to provide every possible information to women, so that they can truly make free, independent and conscious choices. Women can decide which treatments to have during pregnancy (with the local midwives or the gynaecologist or a team of hospital staff), she can choose the type of prenatal care to undergo, the place where to give birth (at home, in a birth centre or hospital) and by whom to receive postnatal care. All these treatments are dependent on the national health system.

XXVIII

Lotus Birth

Lotus Birth is a truly innovative field and, like all innovations, this must be taken with due caution. The revolutionary concept for us is to leave the child connected to the placenta until it spontaneously detaches itself.

The Lotus Birth technique has been developed and theorised for the first time, in recent times, by Australian researcher Shivam Rachana who has recovered very ancient Oriental techniques, but not only.

The placenta is something very complex. It is not at a simple anchor for the umbilical cord and not even a sort of passive "filter" through which the nutrients transit from the mother to the fetus, as many think. The placenta has its own metabolism that regulates maternal functions through the active production of hormones and by selecting the transit of substances from the mother to the child, maintaining the balance between the two and keeping the maternal circulation from the fetal blood, at the same time. It is an extremely intelligent organ, whose function begins after the egg's nesting, at the crucial moment when the embryo protrudes from a sort of bed in the wall of the uterus. This stage is very important. The maternal uterus accepts the fetus, which engages in its own development. It is an intimate and personal event that, nine months later, at the moment of birth, brings us back to this initial event. It is, therefore, a commitment and a fulfilment and can have profound implications in the primary mother-child relationship, constituting its organic base.

The placenta is formed during the first ten weeks of pregnancy and in the third month it is completely ripe. It transmits nutrients to the fetus through the umbilical cord and disposes of the waste: a two-way exchange that takes place through the three large vessels of the umbilical cord.

Cutting the cord means first of all depriving the child of substances and blood supply; moreover, one acts on the emotional sphere of the child with implications related to his future relational life. According to Rachana – and for those who believe in the complexity of subtle bodies that surround every human being – we must also consider what happens on the etheric and energetical.

The Lotus Birth provides all the necessary attention to the child's body, ensuring that he receives all the oxygen-rich and highly nutritious blood that is present in the cord. If the cord is bound tied it ceases to pulsate, the baby does not receive that reserve of blood (from 54 to 160 ml) contained in the placenta; the loss of 30 ml of blood in a newborn is equivalent to the loss of 600 ml in an adult! The common practice of immediately cutting off the cord before the pulsations cease can deprive it of up to 160 ml of blood (the equivalent of a haemorrhagic loss of 1200 ml in an adult), which could explain the strange phenomenon of weight loss in the majority of newborns. The new organism is suddenly subjected to an unnecessary stressful situation caused by having to reproduce the denied blood.

Not only: we should also wonder if the sudden lack of iron-rich cord blood, is not one of the causes of neonatal and childhood anemia.

The placenta helps the immature liver of the newborn to eliminate toxins, as the pumping continues until the pulsation ceases.

The absence of stress from the new organism nourishes the emotional body, which benefits from the uninterrupted supply of oxytocin (the hormone of love) provided by the placenta instead of adrenaline, which comes into operation when survival is in danger. This gives the baby a primary imprint of wellbeing and bliss since the earliest sensory perceptions of lights, sounds, smells and tastes.

When it empties of the blood it contains, the cord takes on the appearance of a beautiful silvery flat ribbon. However, its function still continues, because the vital energy present in the placenta continues to actively transfer to the child, until its aura is complete. In this period, which can last from three to seven days, the cord takes on a brown color and becomes crumbly. When the completion of the aura has occurred, the cord comes off spontaneously from the belly button and at this point, the "Lotus Birth" is over.

Lotus Birth Protocol

Below is a brief "technical" description of the different stages of the Lotus Birth:

1. Wait for the placenta to be expelled naturally; then place it in a basin next to the child.
2. Gently wash the placenta with warm water, removing any remaining blood; delicately absorb any redundant liquid with a cloth.
3. Remember: children like to be informed about what you are doing, even if you think they are not able to understand...
4. The placenta should be wrapped in an absorbent cloth or introduced into a bag to be renewed every day; moisten the cord.
5. Make sure that the distance between the placenta and the child is such that the cord is not stretched.
6. Cover the child with a wide garment, open at the front.
7. If the cord gets dry, it must be moistened to give it its best shape.
8. Do not tighten baby diapers too much; it is better if you lay the child on a small stack of diapers: it will be easier to change them.
9. During all this phase, ensure that the surroundings are as peaceful, serene and silent as possible.

I personally consider this technique to be really extraordinary and I therefore invite you to read the book *Lotus Birth* by Shivam Rachana.

I am however aware of the fact that this technique is a break in today's prevailing patterns, which obliges a mother who really wants to put it into practice, to ask herself whether the pioneer's soul is really in her! Furthermore, an assisting staff ranging from the midwife to the doctor, should be established around the mother and the child, to be able to intervene in the event of any complications.

I like to think that, in a not too distant future, the Lotus Birth technique will rank amongst the most widespread methods, with all the dignity it deserves.

Listen to the sound of the waves
for the Breath of God.
You feel His Voice in the murmur of the Wind.
Find His Teaching of Wisdom in the Earth.
Receive the gift of His Love from the Sun.

Sarasvati

XXIX

Welcoming the child at birth

The welcome to give the child at birth is set against the moment of conception with equal importance and meaning. The following information should be carefully read by everyone, especially doctors, midwives, future mothers, because they are of paramount importance.

First of all, in the delivery room (well-heated room) silence must prevail, the light must be suffused, the presence of people should be reduced to a maximum of three: the mother-to-be, the midwife and the future father, if he wants to participate. A doctor intervenes only if necessary. A sweet background music, chosen by the pregnant woman, can help to create an atmosphere of intimacy suitable for the moment, an intimacy that must be respected in all forms, avoiding any source of potential distraction.

It is known that the instinctive functions that accompany and make labour possible and birth spontaneous are regulated by the primitive brain. While the woman abandons herself to these stimuli, the new part of the brain (the neocortex) should absolutely not be stimulated. Any interference that compels the woman to reason rationally or awaken in her the feeling of being in danger can break the spell. A single disturbance factor can cause the temporary or total interruption of labour, possibly requiring medical and pharmacological interventions and, consequently, prolonging the whole process.

Since the birth path has become medical competence and maternity wards have been created, protocols are applied that immediately imposed the immediate cut of the umbilical cord and the removal of the newborn from the mother, right after birth, to let her rest and run some tests and health checks on the child. These strict rules, applied indiscriminately, can have long-term consequences that are extremely negative on the child and are carefully explained in Primal Health Research.

Fortunately, hospitals and midwives are increasing, updating their protocols based on this data and encouraging the immediate mother-child encounter, which is the right thing. In fact, there are various reasons to respect this moment, to make it become a real sacred event, which is the basis of imprinting, that is, that *imprint* that will exercise its beneficial function throughout life.

I strongly recommend to new mothers to experience these first moments very intensely, because they form a basis for the rest of their existence, to their little one, to themselves and to the whole family. Society will also benefit from this.

As soon as the baby is born, it must be immediately put on the mother's belly, from where the baby will tend towards the mother's breast. At that point, with the umbilical cord still intact, the child is placed in the mother's arms (skin against skin), where mother and child will exchange the first glance, thus experiencing a moment of profound silence and subtle communication. The mother, together with the father, will make a brief rite of presentation, pronouncing loving words of mutual recognition and mutual belonging.

Everyone will externalise the emotions he feels in that solemn moment, a moment that will leave in the child, accepted in that way, an indelible mark for all his life.

At the same time, mother and child secrete a hormone, the oxytocin, also called the "love hormone", which will help them recognise each other and give birth to each other's attachment. This sweet encounter will last until the moment when the placenta will "be born", after which the umbilical cord can be cut (but only where a clear, white area will show). Generally, the cut is performed by the father.

The cut of the umbilical cord requires a lot of attention. The body, which connects the child to the placenta – source of nourishment and all the substances necessary for its growth – belongs to its fetal structure. Therefore, quickly cutting it causes pain similar to that of an amputation. The light area, which is formed at a certain point near the belly button, signifies that the function of the umbilical cord is complete. Only then can it be cut.

When all this does not happen because the newborn, promptly separated from the umbilical cord and wrapped in a cloth, is immediately removed from the delivery room to undergo various examinations and checks, the abrupt detachment from the mother leaves a very painful emptiness in the child.

Try to identify yourself with the situation of a newborn who, at the end of a hard effort to get to the end of that path so narrow and tiring, suddenly finds himself in foreign hands that don't even show it to his mother! (This happened in all the Maternity clinics for tens of years, now, fortunately, things are changing, but still too slowly).

The sudden transition from being a fetus, completely dependent on the mother, to being a newborn, catapulted into an unknown space, takes place within a few minutes. In that short space of time, all the circuits must be renewed in the child's brain to allow him to breathe, suck, see... The change is dramatic, rapid, intense, and at that moment it is only in the loving arms of the mother that the child can feel protected and safe.

Moreover, we must not forget that when the child is born, it still belongs to the world from which it comes, so it must be helped to enter the world of matter gently. And who can help him better than his mother?

After childbirth, mother and child remain a single body (we talk about "eighteen months of pregnancy": nine inside and nine outside), both physically (feeding on breast milk) and in other aspects, just as during gestation. This is why it is important to keep the baby in contact with the mother, day and night.

Moreover, the child, at birth, is enclosed in the mother's energy field (aura), still forming one with her. As long as the child's energy field is not formed around the child, he will have to stay in close contact with his mother as much as possible.

The child's energy field will slowly form during the first months after birth and, when the baby feels ready after being continuously in contact with his mother, he will manifest himself the desire to go ashore to start exploring the world and, when he feels the need, he can then return to his mother, to a mother that is always ready to meet his needs.

Another reason why the newly born baby should not be turned away from the mother is that, if attached to her breast, the baby receives the colostrum. In colostrum, there are high levels of antibodies that help the child defend itself from bacteria that might have been contracted from contact with stranger.

I have not yet described what happens in the course of the child's life, when it was not possible, at the time of birth, to properly welcome the child.

The child, away from his mother, cries and despairs because he feels abandoned. He calls her, but she does not come to help him. This drives the child to desperation, until he stops crying because exhausted and disappointed. "I need my mother so much, but she is not there": this is how the fear of abandonment, anger, hatred, disappointment accumulate in the child's mind... Feelings that will later re-emerge to manifest themselves in the most unusual, even violent forms.

Initially, the child obtains the first self-consolation by inserting the thumb in the mouth, a surrogate of the mother's breast. The mother will replace it with a pacifier. Then follows the strong bond with a stuffed animal, that will be kept close to him day and night. Growing up, the greedy desire for food and sweets will take over; then the smoking, the alcohol... In time, it will discover the drug, first light and then always heavier and so on.

Meanwhile, the years pass and other factors take over, as well as a variety of characteristics that make complicate life for the individual himself and for the people around him. They are all feelings of revenge intended to fill that terrible initial emptiness, that painful split that has remained hidden in the unconscious, but always present.

If the mother, at the time of childbirth, had wanted to fully experience the moment of Imprinting with her partner but, for reasons of *force majeure*, this had not been possible (caesarean section, epidural or other complications) she will be able to fill this gap later. If the mother keeps the child close to her as much as possible, day and night, showing tenderness and intense love, she will succeed at least in part, to fill that terrible initial emptiness, created when it was not possible to do otherwise. The mother will talk to her child telling him everything she wanted to do and her disappointment for what happened. The child will not understand the words, but will grasp that flow of tenderness and love that knows no obstacles. This will avoid, as far as possible, all the harmful consequences for the child, for the family and for society.

Another tip to the future Mothers: in the choice of the clinic where you will give birth, make sure that the protocol contemplates, at the birth of the child, the right treatment, in order not to encounter the issues that I have described. In addition, the baby will have to stay 24 hours a day next to the mother (*Rooming-in*), where she will be able to observe, caress and learn to know, nurturing that strong feeling that will remain alive in both the mother and the child, for life. If the clinic protocol should contemplate different things, do not hesitate to demand what you think is right!

The knowledge of all the details described above and their application on a large scale, could really help to give birth to healthy and balanced creatures, ready for a better life. Future generations, families and society as a whole would benefit.

My religion is loving kindness.

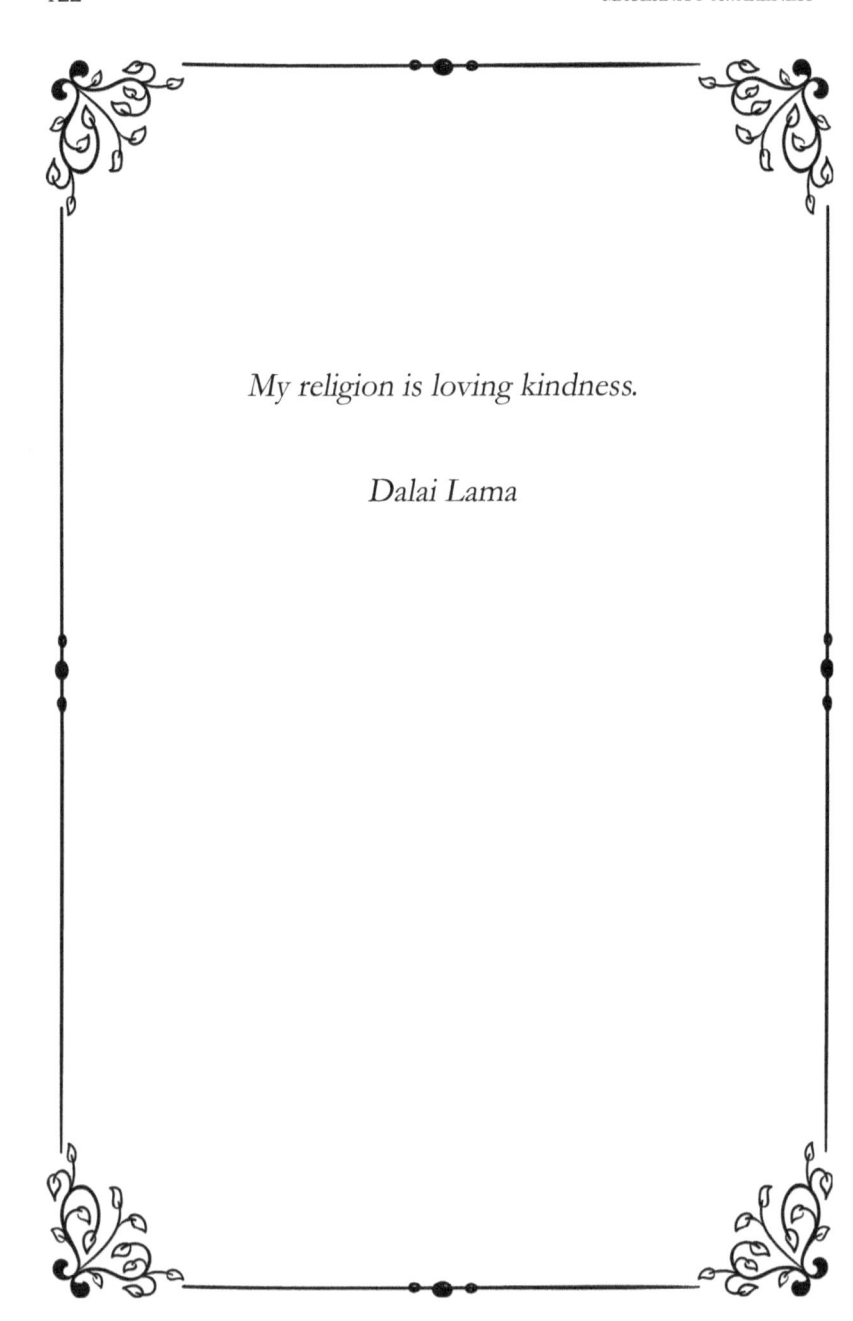

Dalai Lama

XXX

The wound that medicine does not recognise

In some hospitals and maternity clinics, the infant is removed from the mother a few minutes after giving birth "to let her rest". They say this drastic separation, which can even last several hours, without showing the mother the fruit of the long pregnancy, during which the woman just waited for the moment to hold her baby in her arms, also creates a moral wound in the new mother's deep soul.

As if the woman, who was about to give birth, had come to the clinic to let the doctors do their job, and not the other way around! How can a woman who has conceived and grown within herself that child rest away from him, if she has not even had time to see him, to know him, to accept him, to touch him?

From the first moment after birth, the woman needs respect and protection, to establish her relationship with her child. Have you ever observed an animal giving birth? For female mammals, the moment of birth is a very delicate moment. They hide and do not want to be touched or moved, and good luck touching the puppy! If the mother smells a foreign smell, or realises that the puppy has been moved, she often rejects it, with dramatic consequences. The emotions during childbirth are so strong that they do not allow us to reflect on what is really happening so that, in the end, the mother finds herself alone, empty, without the possibility of a physical contact with the creature who she gave birth to.

Birth, which once belonged to the world of women, in which women assisted women, has passed into the hands of the medical world. This has meant, in the last century, the channelling of pregnant women to maternity clinics. On the one hand, this has led to numerous positive aspects (such as the sharp reduction in both female and child mortality, as well as the ability to immediately remedy many diseases or problems) and on the other has led to the loss of all those values that characterise the "coming into the world" of a new being and which should make the birth of a child, a sacred event. Unfortunately, the woman and the child are often treated as impersonal patients and the applied procedures do not take into account the high emotional and intimate value of the birth event: a fundamental experience for family cohesion is thus belittled in the name of safety.

An adequate modification of the protocols would be enough to guarantee a respectful treatment while safeguarding safety! The experience of caring midwives and sensitive doctors such as Michel Odent, demonstrate this to a large extent. Often, the wound that the woman suffers after childbirth awakens past pains, hidden in the unconscious or in the innermost corners of the heart. Pains that can create a strong state of depression, preventing her from feeling love for the newborn baby and for people who would like to help her or, she feels love, but a love tinted with pain. There may also be physical pain but above all profound pain, the emotional suffering of the soul, in the regret of what has been made impossible: the immediate contact with your child. Thus, the woman, instead of feeling joy at the birth of her child, feeling deprived of her innate ability to care for and nurture the bond with her child, feels only sadness and inadequacy.

Like the children, who miss the first contact with their mother and suffer from the lack of expressions of love and psychologically turn off, so the "wounded" mothers, deprived of this joyful experience will hardly be able to be happy and positive mothers. Only a positive start in breastfeeding, can be a means of making contact with your child and starting the healing process.

It should not be forgotten that lack of love inclines to aggression and violence. Basically, like every child at birth needs to be in contact with their mother, every mother after giving birth, needs to be with her child.

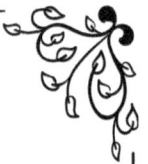

*Nobody can teach you anything
if you do not awaken what in half-sleep
lies in the grass of your conscience.
The teacher who walks
in the shadow of the temple among the disciples
does not give his science
but his love and his faith.
And if he is wise,
he does not invite you to enter
in the house of his science,
but it leads you
to the threshold of your mind.*

Kahlil Gibran

XXXI

Possible disorders during pregnancy

During this journey, a series of disturbances may occur that make pregnancy less pleasant, due to various changes that the female body undergoes. Not all women are the same as not all pregnancies are equal, so for some mothers these problems will be very few and not particularly evident, while for others they will be more accentuated. For each of these there are remedies, but what is effective for one person is not necessarily the same for another. The advice is to experiment, to get to understand what is best for each of us.

Behavioural inconsistencies

Behavioural and mood instability is perhaps one of the hallmarks of pregnancy, due to hormonal changes but also due to the fact that the woman manifests her fears, her insecurities on the progress and on the outcome of pregnancy. Usually these phenomena have a short duration but it is possible that perhaps latent imbalances may occur, which can lead to a real depression. For this reason, it is necessary for the pregnant woman to have the support and closeness of people, who can accompany her in this process of transformation and make her overcome difficult moments.

Nausea and vomit

They can appear around the 4th week up to the 12th-14th week. Although the precise cause is not yet well known, it is hypothesised that these problems are due to hormonal changes or emotional reaction to pregnancy. To prevent them, it is advisable to distribute small meals throughout the day, rather than having a few large meals. Before getting out of bed in the morning you can eat a dry food (crackers, biscuits); movement is always a good solution like a walk in the open air.

Other remedies: eat ginger (root, capsules, candied fruit, biscuits) or drink herbal teas or mint tea. An alternative may be the "anti vomit" bracelets, commonly used for car sickness. You should also try to always be in a comfortable position and do not go to bed immediately after eating.

Pollakiuria

The need to frequently urinate is another rather annoying disorder that may occur during pregnancy. The causes are of nervous, hormonal and mechanical origin, due to the increased volume of the uterus that exerts pressure on the bladder. This disorder usually disappears towards the end of the first trimester but may reappear towards the end of pregnancy, when the baby's head is lowered and then compresses the bladder. The important thing is not to reduce the intake of liquids, which are necessary. One trick would be to not drink too much in the evening, before going to sleep, so that you can sleep without disturbances.

Stomach ache

You may experience a widespread burning in the stomach climbs the oesophagus caused by a decrease in gastric movements. This is mainly due to hormonal causes and stress. It can occur at any time of the pregnancy. It is possible to prevent it with the consumption of vitamins B1 and B2 in order to promote digestive and metabolic functions (brewer's yeast, eggs, pineapple, buckwheat).

As in the case of nausea, it is advisable to consume small meals distributed throughout the day, decrease the consumption of coffee, fat or fried foods, eliminate cigarettes and control posture. Fennel infusions, mint, anise and chamomile can have positive effects.

Constipation

Due to the reduced intestinal peristalsis, a slow rate of excretion may appear from the beginning of pregnancy. It is important to drink plenty of fluids, chew your food well and slowly, consume a good amount of fibre every day (fruit, vegetables, wheat). A nice walk may have a positive effect. Laxatives based on flaxseeds can be used, which form more voluminous faeces and therefore more easily excreted. Other remedies may be dandelion, fennel, flaxseed or plum juice or even glass of warm water on an empty stomach.

Hemorrhoids

During pregnancy, a dilation of the blood vessels occurs due to the compression of the uterus on the blood vessels. In order to avoid them, it is advisable to avoid constipation and intestinal strains and to take vitamin C which has a toning action on the blood vessels (citrus fruits, kiwis, strawberries, green leaves). Once the hemorrhoids have appeared, it is advisable to expose the hemorrhoids to lukewarm water inside a basin as well as the application of propolis or other appropriate ointments.

Varicose veins

They are caused by the thinning and subsequent failure of the diameter of a vein due, to the thinning or lengthening of its walls. The causes are hormonal and mechanical, related to compression of the uterus on blood vessels. The lower limbs, the *labia majora*, the vagina and the uterus can be affected and they are more frequent in those who hold the erect position for a long time. It is important to take Vitamin C and E (sunflower seeds, milk or yogurt – but with moderation – peanuts, wheat germ, walnuts). It would be good to avoid tight clothes that compress and to wear good quality stockings as well as walking often. Avoid standing or sitting too long. Try to rest as much as possible with the feet up and, if you have to stand for a long time, continuously shift the weight from one leg to the other.

Gingivitis and bleeding gums

The accentuated hormonal stimulus facilitates bleeding gums. To tone the walls of the blood vessels, it is advisable to consume Vitamins C and A. It is recommended to use soft, less aggressive toothbrushes.

Backaches

The growth of the fetus affects the future mothers' posture, which requires an adjustment of the ligaments and joints. It is important to practice regular physical activity, avoid lifting weights and, should you weight-lift, doing so by bending the knees and not the back. One must then try to make weight gain regular. Avoid the use high-heeled shoes because they increase the tension on the back. Maintain a proper posture while sitting is important, as is trying to move often and change position. A good massage can help relieve pain and muscle tension.

Cramps

They can occur at any time of pregnancy and the cause is not yet well known. Physical activity is always recommended as when combined with a good consumption of calcium (dairy products, eggs, carrots, almonds, walnuts, green leafy vegetables) and, if necessary, potassium supplements. It is advisable to often change position during the day and to rest by placing a pillow under the legs.

Insomnia

Insomnia especially appears in the third quarter, due to fetal movements, difficulty in finding suitable positions and anxiety. A hot bath may be beneficial before going to bed. It is best to avoid abundant dinners and, above all, avoid coffee. Experiment with different positions, with the help of pillows. A hot herbal tea, a good book and soft lighting can help.

XXXII

Post-partum depression

This is a topic that I would like to avoid discussing, because it casts a shadow of sadness on an event that I would like to continue believing to be a bearer of joy and gratification. However, the frequency with which episodes due to depression occur are now growing and, at least in the West, too numerous to be neglected. It is estimated that 20% of Western women are affected, compared to 10% in the rest of the world.

In our society every parent, especially the mother, creates important expectations after the birth of the child, often too high and in conflict with their own strength, with their position in society, with the economic possibilities, with their role in the couple. All of this is very anxiety-inducing. We have not yet learned to grant ourselves permission to rest and to ask for help when we need it.

Post-partum depression is a pathology that is often not recognised, neglected, unexpected, set aside by both the woman herself and her family members as well as by medical professionals. A depressive state is perceived as unlikely after a successful birth, when there is happiness for the event and the whole family is serene.

A woman narrates:

After the birth of my child I understood that something was wrong with me. I felt detached from everything, I had bizarre thoughts, numerous physical symptoms such as feeling cold, shaking and feeling insensitive. When I was alone at home these symptoms increased. I cried often when someone spoke to me. I had no appetite, I could not sleep. I was terrified by anxiety, I had panic attacks. I felt out of control and I was afraid of going crazy.

First of all, let's clarify the terms. There is a "puerperal crisis" that occurs in more than 50% of cases. This should not alarm you: it may last from the third day up to two weeks after delivery. In this crisis the woman feels tired, exhausted and more prone to crying. These symptoms do not last long and the causes are due to strong hormonal variations (often sudden prolactin peaks) and emotional variations. The "puerperal crisis" should not be confused with the more serious post-partum depression.

There is also a "puerperal psychosis", a serious psychosomatic disease, that fortunately appears in only 1 or 2 cases in 1000, which requires immediate hospitalisation and a psychopharmacological drug therapy as well as constant 24-hour monitoring of the patient.

Lastly, there is the post-partum depression. Those who suffer from it begin to feel their symptoms a few days after giving birth but more intensely from the sixth week onwards. There are also those who fall into depression much later, often many months after giving birth.

Mothers may be victims during the first, but also the second or third pregnancy experience. A woman who has experienced post-partum depression after her first child is likely to experience the depression again, in the following pregnancies. If not treated promptly and appropriately, this depression can evolve into something devastating, both for the woman, the child and the whole family balance.

The subtle aspect is that the woman, after giving birth, tends to avoid giving importance to alarming symptoms because she lives them with a sense of guilt at a time that should be devoted to happiness. Sometimes, *post-partum* depression hides behind symptoms such as tiredness, instability, sadness and whining; everything seems tiring, there is little energy and little motivation, a sense of inadequacy for new needs and often lack of concentration. If neglected, these alarm bells light up, turning into anxiety and triggering a dangerous spiral. Therefore, do not keep the symptoms secret from your partner, your midwife, your gynaecologist or your pediatrician.

What is the origin of post-partum depression? There are various theories, which can coexist in the same case, even if to different extents...

- "Organic" origin. The hormonal variations (oestrogen, progesterone etc.) are very intense and sudden after deliver but can be easily controlled by the doctor. The ongoing studies on other possible organic causes will most likely surprise us: we are expecting a great deal of research to ascertain the relationship between *post-partum* depression, vitamin and oligo-element deficiency.

- "Relational" origin. The child often becomes a symbol, an opportunity to fill inconclusive emotional experiences; as if to say that in this period many wounds of the past come to the surface. In this case, expectations, whether own or of others, become excessive and therefore cause disappointment.

A medical anamnesis aimed at investigating whether depressive episodes, whether related to birth or not, have already occurred is very useful. It is also important to check if a "history" of depressions or polarity disorders exist within the family.

In traditional Chinese culture, special food and complete care is guaranteed to the mother, after giving birth, for forty days. Chinese medicine recognises that, after giving birth, the mother becomes "cold": she therefore needs heat on all levels. Protection is very meticulous because it is believed that diseases, the future physical and psychological problems of these women will depend on how they spend those first, delicate forty days.

The partners of depressed mothers often confess of feeling frightened and confused, unable to improve a situation that escapes their comprehension. Feeling surprised by the different attitude of the partner who became a mother, sometimes, even the terror that the situation can last over time, foreshadowing negative consequences. Even these partners should be given therapeutic help, normally of psychological nature.

Women suffering from post-partum depression must be able to freely express the emotions they experience that are commonly experienced by many other women, to be attentively listened to, to realise what is happening to them and not to feel guilty. In these cases, help can come from a friend who is available to give time and comfort, possibly a person who has lived and been through the same experiences, which can then better understand their situation. The important thing, in these cases, is to intervene promptly.

The role of the partner is fundamental, both in recognising the symptoms and in liaising with the doctors. Since this depression is a phenomenon that manifests itself in 1 every 5 cases, it is logical that the man should be appropriately informed regarding the importance of managing this situation properly.

What do you think makes the Earth turn
if not Love?
And what do you think the fire of your Sun is made of,
and the cells of your body
and the stars of your Sky
and the knowledge of your Heart?

Everything is LOVE.

Emmanuel

XXXIII

The breastfeeding

Mum, your milk contains more than love...

Breastfeeding is a very important phase in the life of the child and the mother. For the newborn, attaching to the breast and sucking does not only represent the satisfaction of a primary physiological need, but it represents a moment of deep relationship and connection with the mother, rich in emotions and tactile, acoustic, taste and olfactory sensations. The satisfaction of this need procures both a profound sense of well-being and tranquillity. The resulting consequences enrich both the mother and the child but at the same time, the whole society.

Breastfeeding offers a wonderful opportunity for mother and child to get to know each other right from the first hours after birth. Breast milk production and lactation are the natural continuation of pregnancy and childbirth. In fact, the sequence of reproduction includes conception, pregnancy, birth and lactation.

Pregnancy, childbirth and breastfeeding characterize a particular phase of a woman's life that brings with her a series of extraordinary emotions. Breast-feeding mothers find this to represent inner fulfilment: it is the completion of their nature as a woman in the awareness of giving their child the most natural and most appropriate food.

In the first period of life, breast milk is an irreplaceable food for the newborn. In fact, it presents specific characteristics that don't only differ from species to species, but also from child to child. The milk of women who have given birth to a pre-term child has a higher protein content than that of women whose birth has regularly been completed.

Breast milk is the only source of important elements that help protect the infant's immune system during its development. In fact, antibodies, specific to the environment in which they live, are transmitted to the baby through the mother's milk.

As research into the composition of breast milk is deepened, one realises how perfect this food is and which makes the mother a loving nurse. In fact, it has been shown that breast milk is a food that is suitable for the digestive system of the developing baby and contains: proteins, fat, calcium, phosphorus, potassium, iron, copper, zinc and vitamins D, E, C and K, all in the correct proportions that are useful for the gradual growth of the child. The mother must therefore take care of properly feeding herself in order to better feed her child.

The contemporary medical and psychological literature is in full agreement on the superiority of breastfeeding compared to every other form of feeding of the newborn and the child in the early evolutionary phases. When the mouth eagerly sucks the milk from the nipple, the child practices an exercise that will serve to develop the jaw and facial structure appropriately, which will affect the ability to smile and, subsequently, to speak clearly, avoiding at the same time orthodontic problems. Furthermore, breastfeeding inclines the newborn to the maintenance of a normal weight, a guarantee against the future tendency towards obesity.

In breastfeeding done with love, milk, full of emotions, transmits to the child those extraordinary etheric particles that make nutrition a complete energetic function. In fact, the mother's milk feeds the child's body, but also his mind, thus giving birth to the need to relate to the mother. Moreover, from a psychological perspective, the mother-child physical contact leads to reinforcing the union between the two.

The newborn has only three needs: the warmth of the mother's arms, the milk of her breasts and the mother's safety, needs that maternal breastfeeding fully satisfies.

In short words...

Here is a brief summary of the main benefits of breastfeeding for the newborn...

- Breast milk is the ideal and inimitable food due to its easy tolerability and digestibility;
- It is also a natural immune defence system, thanks to the presence of antibodies and therefore prevents infections and allergies;
- Body growth is more regular (and there is less tendency to get fat);

- Newborns are calmer and sleep more, as well as making mothers sleep more for the production of prolactin;
- Studies show that breastfed babies are less likely to get sick from certain diseases even in adulthood.

... and for the mother ...

- Better relationship with the newborn;
- Immediately after delivery, due to the mammillo-hypothalamic reflex, the contraction and a faster involution of the uterus occurs, with the consequent reduction of blood loss;
- After a few months, return to the pre-pregnancy weight due to the greater consumption of calories;
- Reduction of risk of breast cancer and of other organs of the genital sphere;
- Convenience and practicality: milk is always available and, in every place, you do not need to prepare anything.

Weaning occurs gradually and spontaneously. When the child feels that he no longer needs the substances he is looking for in his mother's milk, it is the child himself that stops breastfeeding. Sometimes this occurs even after two years or more. Even the evening suck, before going to sleep, should become part of the "good night ritual". The baby will certainly sleep more peacefully and calmly.

XXXIV

The weaning

The introduction of solid food represents the beginning of a new era in the child-mother-environment interaction and induces the start of a food education project that will also have repercussions much later in the years. It is not a period that is always easy, but not even dramatic. Weaning, in fact, is not to be understood as a drastic interruption of breastfeeding, but as a period in which breastfeeding becomes an addition to the baby food. Slowly and gradually proposing new foods and simultaneously maintaining the supply of breast milk, the child will be able to get used to without abrupt changes to new foods and their digestion.

Breastfeeding ceases when the child decides it. There are children who do not want to be breast-fed at eight months, while others continue for much longer. The child is "the pediatrician of himself" and knows his physiology well, by instinct.

Nowadays we know that if the child prolongs the demand for breast milk, it is because he still needs it and it needs to intake some substances that complete the development of the nerve sheaths of the hypothalamus phospholipids. It is therefore thought, that if the child continues to request breast milk even after the year of age, he does so to achieve a precise maturation of his central nervous system, as claimed by Lorenzo Braibanti, Italian pioneer of birth without violence and natural breastfeeding.

During weaning, the child explores the specific characteristics of new foods with lips, teeth, smell, palate (flavour, consistency, smell, warmth), knows with the eyes (shape and color) and with the touch; every food strikes and triggers knowledge that is learned and remains in the memory.

In order not to limit and mortify the sensorial vivacity of the child at this particular moment, it is important to have patience. Food remains full of meanings and symbols, but at the same time it must be characterised above, all as an answer to the punctual and ever more differentiated need to eat.

If the introduction of solid foods into the diet is gradual and above all, not in conflict with breastfeeding, in the sense that it does not overthrow it and automatically provokes its disappearance, the child will live this new phase much more comfortably. Even your body will get used to receiving solid nutrients, while breast milk will become increasingly complementary. Studies show that the mother's milk also changes when it is flanked by the new diet, continuing that adjustment based upon the needs of the child.

A child who has not thoroughly experienced the period of breastfeeding – because he was weaned too early or because his mother was unable/unwilling to breastfeed – is likely to face growth with less security. During growth, the child shows that he is ready for new experiences; each, according to his individuality, proceeds by attempts. We need to give it confidence, pay attention to his rejections and his preferences and let him taste as well as enabling him to express his taste.

It is therefore quite understandable, why Mother Nature has established everything for the good of the new creatures that come into the world.

Skin

it is the most extensive sense organ.
The sense of touch is activated very early
because the child is surrounded and caressed
by a warm fluid
and from soft fabrics
from the beginning of fetal life.
Babies love contact, heat
and pleasant surfaces.

John H. Kennel

XXXV

How to carry a child on yourself

Just like plants and animals, that know what they need or what they need to do in order to grow, so does every baby. Every baby knows what is important for their well-being, by instinct. This knowledge is contained in its genes and corresponds to the experience made during intrauterine life.

During gestation, the baby is constantly in contact with the mother: is cradled, massaged and fed through the organs responsible for this function.

After delivery, the newborn expects that the same conditions will continue; therefore, it is very important to meet the baby's expectations. After nine months of warmth, swinging and intimacy with their mother, every child feels a real need, at birth, to stay in touch with her.

Long strips of cloth are available on the market to keep the baby constantly in contact. Being always with the mother, the child feels comfortable and has the opportunity to observe everything he sees doing, learning many things.

For the mother, one of the advantages offered by wearing the baby is to be able to continue to carry out any daily activity. By simply carrying the child on the arm, would impede every movement.

If the child is satisfied in its need to not be abandoned, it instils a feeling of trust in the child: he feels he can count on his parents, a very important feeling for a joyful and balanced growth. This need will last only as long as the child himself makes it clear that he wants to start walking. If you give your child, from the first moment, all he needs, a solid base will be formed in him, upon which he can develop a quiet and independent existence.

> Jacqueline narrates:
>
> *Since Kim was born, I have always carried my baby on my body, supported by this strip of cloth, and I found myself very well. It is very comfortable to use, in every sense. My hands were free and the baby could sleep or participate in my business. Today, I always take Kim with me and carry her on my back, in my backpack, and from that position she has a lot of fun.*

XXXVI

Education

The "continuum" of human life begins with the various stages of prenatal life, and then continues with appropriate methods and teachings in the following stages.

Human life must be considered an indivisible "continuum" in which each of the phases of development is equally important and whose levels are interdependent with each other and are not separable.

In this continuum, the individual represents an indivisible entity, which includes all the functions of his organism at physiological, biochemical, endocrinological and psychological level. It is not possible to separate any of the levels of human development, from the rest of the continuum of the life of the individual. The continuum of life is one of the basic needs of human life, in order to maintain the balance between the various functions.

The importance of the individual's family history is becoming increasingly evident. In fact, the life of the individual begins in the home of the ancestors, of the grandparents, who have transmitted – or have not transmitted – to their children (the current future parents) the basic values of ethics, empathy, respect for life, of gratitude, children who, in turn, will transmit – or will not transmit – these values to their offspring even before it is conceived, to their child in pregnancy and later.

The continuum of human life therefore begins already before birth, to be prolonged with the same care and kindness in all subsequent phases. This means that taking care of conception, pregnancy, childbirth and breastfeeding is a duty that, thanks to what science and psychology taught us, we are aware that the benefits are at on all levels; but this is only the starting point. We must continue after birth through childhood, adolescence and beyond, until the individual is able to stand on his own feet in society with dignity, alone, thanks to the guidance received from the parents.

Let us now read this beautiful excerpt from www.attachmentparenting.eu:

> *Exercising the function of parents in a natural way means teaching empathy through a positive, non-authoritarian disciplinary approach. Children in general should be treated and guided in a respectful manner, respecting them to the same degree that you want to be respected by them. Your children need you for their survival and must see in you a model to learn from. This means that you must be strong and convincing, but flexible at the same time. We are alarmed to see the distance that is being created between the world of children and the adult world. If we want our children to get a realistic view of the world, we must offer them the chance to share it with us.*

Now, the habit of keeping the little ones always with oneself, day and night, is spreading quickly among the mothers, until the moment when the child expresses the need to move more freely. It is then that the task of guiding him into everything he wants to do is commences, not with strict orders, but always explaining why one can do or cannot do a certain thing, and how to proceed without causing any damage.

In this way, you can introduce the child to many aspects of daily life, teaching certain values such as respect for mum and dad, for all people, for the environment in which it is located, for food, for objects, for the animals, for plants, for nature in general, always giving signs of approval for every gesture made in the right way.

It would be nice to be able to explain to every child that everything must be respected because, in a certain sense, every apparently static object has life and meaning. It can be appreciated, because it is useful, because it is beautiful, because it reminds a loved one or for many other reasons. However, everything must be respected.

Even the teaching of certain rules is essential, rules that must be formulated according to the character of the child. This way of educating generates full trust in the parents because they feel they are guided well and taken on a dignified path.

I think it is very useful and important also to teach to feel gratitude for all that they receive, gratitude that leads to empathy.

It is natural that the child of all ages should be left free to move, to experience everything. Constriction must not exist: this can be eliminated by giving simple but convincing explanations. When the child perceives that what he is told is solely for his own good, listen.

Naturally, the task of education is not limited to what has been said. It is up to those who constantly follow the child to understand it and adapt to its characteristics. Each child has personal qualities that must be respected and left free to take shape according to natural trends.

In essence, every child must have full freedom of action, reasoning and thought, but under a constant and loving guidance that makes him understand that there are limits. These are necessary to help them become balanced people. People who have learned not to hurt people or things because they have learned respect.

Only by proceeding in this way will we raise those creatures that the world so badly needs. Giving importance to the phase preceding birth is important but not sufficient. We must continue with a careful and loving education, adapted to the various ages, which satisfies all the emotional and intellectual needs, to build the adult of the future.

Only on the basis of a wise and loving education can we create a better world. Finally, let us always remember: there is no education without freedom, just as there is no freedom without education.

XXXVII

The mystery, the creation, the sacredness

We are immersed in a great creative cosmic energy. To date, no science can explain to us exactly why a giant sequoia of more than a hundred meters grows from a seed as big as an olive kernel.

For a believer, it is the work of God, for an atheist or an agnostic it is the result of nature. For all of us a great unsolved mystery. This applies to all the things in the world in which we are immersed, even a simple stone represents in itself a true mystery. Originally it was lava, then solidified. A pile of different elementary materials fused together, whose shape, for example in the case of a river pebble, is given by the forces of nature. Think of the trees that absorb carbon dioxide from the air and give us oxygen, so important for our existence.

The energy that underlies Creation is always the same and it is expressed in infinite forms. Everything that surrounds us, from the diamond to the most common object, originates from creative energy. Animal, vegetable and mineral kingdom, everything! In terms of the birth event, we like to link these considerations to the birth and formation of a new human life.

Nature has given to the woman, to the future mother, with the contribution of the future father, the gift of giving birth to her child. A wonderful fact, a living child, beautiful, perfect and working in all its organs. The mother lacks detailed knowledge of all the organs, their position and their functioning but the work is done on time thanks to the universal creative energy.

I do not expect these considerations to be inventive but I believe that they should lead us to a reconsideration of the created world, as something that is due to immense respect and consideration.

Many wise figures, originating from most diverse cultures, have spoken of the sacredness of nature. I like this concept too. It applies to believers and non-believers, it unites us in a condition of respect, almost of veneration.

Indeed, sacredness which means respect, is an invitation to an attitude of attention, consideration, love and gratitude. The sacredness of all things: a theme that would be most appropriate to teach children! It is not just ecology, or respect for the Earth as a habitat or resource, it is much, much more.

XXXVIII

Conclusion

The woman was given all the requisites to perform, in the best way and at all levels, the role of parent, to become the "Mother of Humanity". In fact, the evolution of the human race depends on the commitment and the spirit with which it carries out its extraordinary function.

In order to be driven by the best understanding in carrying out maternity, not only on the basis of new knowledge, but of a real awakening, it would be necessary for the woman to find in herself the awareness of being the custodian of the role given to her by Nature.

In the last decades of the last century, following a gesture of rebellion, the woman set in motion the recapturing of the position that it deserves in society but a change of this magnitude, requires the assistance of future generations. Even the Men will have a long way to go before finding the right balance in the man-woman relationship, in which everyone is aware of their role, in mutual respect. Since even men have been given a precise task, the two parts will have to become capable of integrating.

In order to have her values recognised and the concept of her inferiority compared to the male world, the woman is demonstrating her skills in all the fields she employs, fields that have nothing to do with motherhood. In fact, she is already successfully occupying positions in society that were once exclusively reserved to men. As a result, the concept of "motherhood" has slipped into the background. The birth rate has significantly dropped compared to the past and even the time to give birth to a child is often postponed until after the deadline.

In the future, thanks to the findings of science and psychology regarding the birth event, the importance of the childbirth event will become widespread and accepted on a larger scale and then, the leap in quality may occur. Only in this way can woman acquire the awareness of their true position in society, that of Mother and the competent Institutions will be willing to give women all the necessary support in terms of time and means to be able to raise and educate their children in complete serenity. Society will benefit from this by having healthy individuals both in the body and mind, capable of demonstrating their moral qualities and their efficiency in cooperating in all fields, for the greater good of the community.

For now, women must be supported in their most immediate task, which is not only to bring children into the world, but also to act, within the family, within society and within any environment and demonstrate love, care, desire to educate, unity, protection, tolerance, consolation and assistance.

It is hoped that all the knowledge that science and psychology have accumulated, from the beginning of research, on everything concerning the birth of a child, will soon be elaborated and shared in the form of a "Procreation Card". It will be important for women and the medical world to take advantage of new guidelines for future births.

The moment will come, when the press will talk about it, there will be training courses for parents and teachers and the theme of procreation will become part of educational programmes at all levels, including universities, so that not only will newly graduates in gynaecology be informed but young people, in general, will know the values that are part of life.

A widespread preparation in this sense would be useful from various points of view:
- Physiological, because it aspires to create healthy individuals;
- Psychological, because it aims to the shaping of the mind of the individual as well as of strong and balanced characters;
- Anthropological, because it is of paramount importance for the future life of humanity and its evolution;
- Prevention, the experience of a happy and serene pregnancy facilitates childbirth, avoids mental traumas and pre-term births, as well as eradicating violence and crime.

Lastly, it would be desirable for this important knowledge to be supported by an authoritative voice, by a luminary in the field of gynaecology in order to spread the information in a more convincing and credible way.

Let us now focus on the need for information: its dissemination would have the aim of laying the foundations for a better quality of life in favour of future generations, society in general and the whole world, taking into account that conception, pregnancy and childbirth constitute the basis of the whole existence of the individual.

This is the reason why they should be treated in the best way, respecting recent discoveries, without however underestimating the importance of education that, after birth, should be given with the same dose of kindness.

We must, however, admit that in this extraordinary work, in which the mother offers her body and all the substances necessary for the formation of the child, an ancient matrix intervenes which, thanks to her collaboration and the intervention of the same energies that have made all Creation possible, gives the following "result": a healthy, intelligent, beautiful and perfect baby in all its details. Is this not a miracle? Does it not deserve to be seen as a "sacred event"?

Consequently, while the woman is pregnant, she should realise that she is a true Helper of the Cosmic Forces, to ensure the continuity of the species. With respect for these Forces, pregnancy should be lived impeccably from all points of view, so that the Cosmic Order of things is not disturbed in the slightest, and the birth of a creature ready to perform in the best way, is achieved.

At this point, it would be advisable to take a quick look at the various stages of the birth event, lit by this new Light. New, compared to when, about pregnancy, little was known and women were unaware of everything.

In summary...

Conception

To become parents together.

Bringing a child into the world is a decision that must be taken in common agreement, that is when both future parents feel ready for many renunciations and ready to adapt to the radical change that takes place with the presence of a new family member. Nevertheless, aware of the great joy they will encounter, capable of abolishing any inconvenience.

At the basis of conception lies Love for the desired child, who must be imagined, dreamed and loved even before knowing it.

Pregnancy

The pregnant woman must know that the nine months of waiting for the child are not an illness and that Nature has provided her with a body able to sustain, from the beginning to the end, any slight discomfort caused by this function.

However, let us remember that: "To give birth to a healthy and strong son in the body, free in the mind and good in feelings, it will be like entering a harmonious note in the great universal symphony".

Labour and delivery

Depending on the interpretation that is given to pain, it can be said that the more a meaning is attributed to it, the higher the threshold of tolerability is raised.

To give a positive interpretation to the pain of labour and childbirth means, however, to transform this phase and to live it actively, as an opportunity for growth and not as a condemnation.

Reception of the child at birth

The welcoming to give to the child at the moment of birth is set against the moment of conception with equal importance and meaning.

There is a very precise process to be followed, of which every detail must be scrupulously respected, so that it does not create the premise for harmful consequences for oneself and for society that could arise in the course of the individual's existence.

In the delivery room, however, immediately removing the child from the mother must be absolutely avoided; the sudden removal of the child from the mother creates in the mind of both a very painful and hard to heal wound that, in the course of life can give rise to very negative consequences and behaviours.

Breastfeeding

The production of breast milk and lactation are the natural continuation of pregnancy and childbirth; in fact, lactation is healthy in the sequence of reproduction. Breastfeeding is a function that enhances femininity. The resulting consequences do not only enrich the mother and child in first person, but at the same time, the whole society.

To conclude, let us now read and understand Leonardo da Vinci's wise words:

Immerse your soul in the divine unconscious, sprouting yourself in it: this is how I have always tried to express my art. My soul became one with this impulse, and from this embrace the expression was born.

Why don't we not apply Leonardo's secret to all the functions of life?

Let's try to imagine a woman waiting for a child. Allowing oneself, during every day of the pregnancy, a moment of concentration to immerse one's soul in the divine unconscious, relying completely on it. One's soul would become one with this impulse and, from that moment, a perfect creature would be born on all levels, with the most positive qualities to build a better world. To be able to immerse oneself in this particular function, however, the woman must first develop in herself the awareness of the role that Nature has entrusted her with and the certainty of being able to live up to it. The woman was given all the requisites to perform, in the best way and on all levels her role as a mother, to become the "Mother of Humanity". The evolution of the human race depends on the way and the spirit with which it carries out this extraordinary function.

Conception, gestation, childbirth, the welcome and lactation: everything should be done by connecting one's soul to the divine unconscious. Thus, the best results would be obtained for the benefit of all.

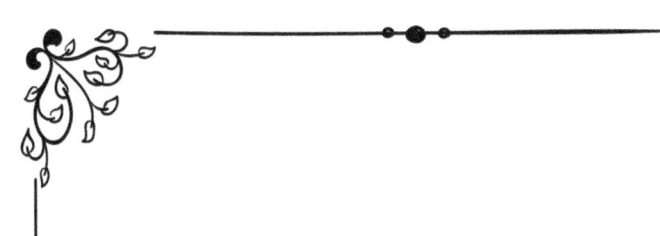

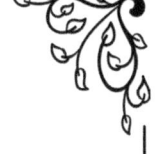

Love's energy:
fundamental principle of the Universe.

David Bohm

XXXIX

The love

The love felt at the beginning, which later turns into a profound pleasure of being together, is kept alive on the basis of some important reflections.

Firstly, it is advisable to understand that:

- Marriage is the union of two beings who chose each other, to integrate and protect one another and to grow and build together, on various levels, a life full of interests and exchanges;
- In marriage, a joyful and harmonious coexistence is based on mutual respect and mutual trust.

Neither of them is superior or inferior to the other. Everyone has his own specific role to play. One needs the other.

XL

Conclusive reflections

So far, I have shared with you the basics of all the important things to know when you want to have a baby. Anyone wishing to know more, you will find on my website www.gravidanzaconsapevole.org / www.maternityawareness.org other interesting scientific and psychological information about the child, both before and after birth. You may also download, for free, an introductory course to pregnancy.

However, there are various things that must always be kept in mind. Here is a final summary...

- Love is the foundation on which a positive birth is based;
- As the French doctor J. P. Relier writes: «Love, whose influence cannot yet be fully measured, is undoubtedly the most appropriate stimulating environmental for the growth and the harmonious balance of a quality being»;
- In every woman, there already is the knowledge of how to give birth to her child;
- A woman in labour needs a serene environment that assures her: intimacy, autonomy and freedom of expression of her emotions and her own needs;

- Every woman faces labour in her own way. One must only help her to trust herself and her body through the mind-body-spirit integration;
- The birth of a child is one of the greatest challenges that life offers: the opportunity for personal growth. Every birth is unique;
- It is important to follow a course of "Preparation to pregnancy and preparation for childbirth" in which mum, dad and child can benefit from extraordinary moments of openness towards a new consciousness, a new awareness that opens to the true values of life, eradicating at the same time, fears and uncertainties.

In essence, my desire is to accompany both parents along the entire path of birth: from before conception to childbirth and beyond, in order to give them the basis to listen to life, to find out who they are and who is their child, and to know what their common commitment as mother and father will be.

I would like all parents to know all the good that can be done for their child starting from before conception. This "good" will benefit the family and society in the future.

I therefore ask all of you to help me spread this important message.

*On a final note, I leave you with three "simple" and deep
reflections written by great thinkers ...*

*If all women were aware
of their potential,
in fifty years
all of humanity could be renewed.*

Omraam Mikhaël Aïvanhov

*Physical, mental and moral health
of the citizen is the basis on which
the happiness and strength of a nation is formed.*

Benjamin Disraeli

*We ourselves must be the change
we want to see in the world.*

Gandhi

Appendix

Appendix 1

A PROJECT FOR THE FUTURE OF HUMANITY

I cannot deny it. When it comes to problems concerning pregnancy, birth and new methods, I become very enthusiastic.

The real spring, after several hints, occurred in me in the eighties, when, by chance, I happened to read one of the writings of Omraam Mikhaël Aïvanhov, translated from French. In fact, the title was: Education begins before birth.

From that moment on I started a studying the subject and at the end of 1992, I entered the world of prenatal education. Congresses, conferences, events and publications have encouraged me to dive into this extremely fascinating world, without ever losing the desire to cultivate what I now consider a mission and a reason for living.

Here is the excerpt which, in my opinion, constitutes the heart of the principle to which I have been inspired and it is for this reason that I launch an appeal to women in the whole world:

> *"Wake up to the awareness of the task that God has entrusted to you. You are the custodians of wonderful secrets, thanks to which you would be able to regenerate humanity but you do not realise it and play with these secrets... Become aware of your mission immediately so that you can carry out this magical work in peace".* Nature has given the woman

powers she does not use or uses badly; it is necessary that she should become aware of it and realise that all the future of mankind depends on it. If all the women of the world want to understand me, they will constitute an immeasurable power; nothing can oppose them. But they will have to unite with each other to aim for a wonderful ideal. [...]

Now all the women of the Earth must unite with each other, with the will to regenerate humanity. In spite of their intelligence and their abilities, men cannot do great things in this field. It is to the woman, to the mother, who has been entrusted with this mission, precisely because nature has given her the ability to influence the child to be born. That is why I ask you to become aware of this great mission of yours and to enlighten other women in the world, who are still unaware of their gifts. This ideal, this desire to be useful will fill your heart, soul and spirit.

You will always feel inspired, always rich, because this ideal of contributing to the happiness of humanity will support you, it will nourish you. As long as you do not bring this ideal into your life, nothing will satisfy you; whatever you possess or do, you will always be in the same state of emptiness, of dissatisfaction.

Only the concern to fulfil the mission that God has entrusted to you, and to do in the best possible way all that Heaven expects of you, will make you radiant, luminous and happy.

Omraam Mikhaël Aïvanhov

Appendix 2

MEDITATION DURING PREGNANCY

Let us now read the beautiful meditation published on the website evelynedisseau.blogspot.com:

Meditating during pregnancy is beautiful!
The future mother who understands the importance of this meditation will derive from this state a physical and mental benefit and will thus be in complete union with her baby in utero.
Nothing could be easier: the future mother, whom I will call "mum", because she is technically already one, sits comfortably in an armchair or wherever she wants, but the important thing is that she is comfortably seated, semi lied down so that there is room for the child to lie down too. (Yes, even the baby in the stomach lies down...). Important: make sure that the phones and mobile phones are switched off and that they do not have physiological needs. Turn music on in the background, such as Mozart's Concerto No. 21 or any favourite music that is relaxing.
Once she is in this position, she closes her eyes, the mother brings her attention to the breath and waits for it to become calm and regular. The body slowly relaxes and abandons itself to the position, hands gently resting on the bench. The jaw is relaxed, the eyelids too. Now Mum feels calm. It may be that the baby is awake makes himself be noticed. Softly, the mother strokes the child with her hands and listens to her movement under her hands. Whether the child moves or not, there is nothing other than this mother-child union in the

present moment. The mother is shown with her child in a soft sphere, colored or not, very bright, and simply observes her feelings.

When this moment ceases to be "magical" and suspended in time, the sphere vanishes. Then the mother takes deep breaths and with her fingers she makes lightly taps her stomach to greet the baby. After stretching the legs, the arms, she yawns and calmly resumes her activities. It is the first level of meditation. It seems easy, but it's not that straight forward because you need to learn to get thoughts out of your head to be able to enter the magical sphere! If the meditation is successful, the mother feels relaxed and recharged and the child rejoices in his mother's state of mind...

Appendix 3

How many ultrasounds can I do?

Going to get an ultrasound after starting the pregnancy is a moment that triggers deep emotions.

Being able to see the child in the strangest positions and in his movements, is truly a gift offered to us by technology. There's really a baby! It is still very small but it is there. The father can also finally see it.

Who would not want to continue to enter the world of the nascent child and monitor him in his evolution?

At this point, however, one must reflect and not let one's curiosity prevail but rather ask oneself whether this intrusion, so desired by the parents, is pleasing to the child.

Does the child hear it?
Of course, and he is not at all happy.

Everyone recommends not to keep the phone in your pocket and not even keep it close to your ear, because the waves that it emanates can be harmful. Even TV watched for a long time, especially by children, can affect health. How can the waves emitted by the ultrasound, which are very loud and noisy, not disturb such a delicate and small creature?

What is the ultrasound examination for? Here are the answers...

After the first trimester:

- To establish the number of fetuses;
- To date the pregnancy based on the length of the fetus;
- To verify the vitality of the fetus and the cardiac activity;
- To signal uterine or adnexal anomalies.

After the second trimester:

- To evaluate the anatomy of the fetus (measure head, abdomen and femur);
- To assess the amount of amniotic fluid and the positioning of the placenta.

After the third trimester:

- To evaluate the growth of the fetus;
- To evaluate the amount of amniotic fluid and the positioning of the placenta.

The scientific community recommends not to exaggerate with the use of the ultrasound: exaggerating would imply a promotion of medical consumerism. Rather, it is orienting itself in recommending no more than three, or rather, only two ultrasounds: an initial one for the screening of chromosomal malformations and the other to be carried out towards the twentieth week, for a general control.

This naturally applies to a normal pregnancy, while for women with problems (diabetes, kidney disease, hypertension or the use of certain drugs), it may be appropriate to do a greater number of checks.

More and more mothers ask the gynaecologist for a "souvenir photo" – this has become a fashion. Please do not let yourself be caught by this "whim": it would be a lack of respect towards your child.

Appendix 4

It is cruel to let children cry

What does a baby need? Not just food but physical contact with the mother... a skin contact, smell, heat... it is not by chance that smell is the first indicators that newborns recognise their mother. Above all, with the research for the mother's breast, the child instinctively strives to obtain both physical and emotional nourishment, to satisfy the need for security with the confirmation that he will not be abandoned.

Let's put ourselves in the child's shoes, whose brain has been programmed for millenniums to be in contact with his mother, the only one that can guarantee tranquillity. It is precisely the contact with the mother that gives the little one, beyond the food, the deepest well-being: the trust of being loved and the certainty of having a secure base.

In the very small child, that is emotionally very complex, the separation anxiety panic immediately activates the crying. Unfortunately, a solid strand of the psychology of the evolutionary age continues to affirm that if the child has been breastfed, changed and cuddled, when he is put in his crib he has no reason to cry; if he cries, it is out of sheer whim, and to avoid spoiling him, you have to let him cry, so he learns to feel good by himself, stoically closing his bedroom door ...

In contrast to this absurd statement, it should be emphasised that in newborns there are no whims. Crying is the only means of expression, the mother or the one who usually takes care of the baby learns to recognise, according to the type of crying, what is the baby's need at that moment. It can be hunger, thirst, heat, cold or need to cuddle, to be cleaned or even just turned. Every need is expressed with a type of crying and every call must be indulged as soon as possible to give the child the sensation of having launched a signal that makes sense. In this case, the child becomes confident and remains calm. If, on the other hand, you repeatedly let it cry for a long time, the baby thinks that he has made only unnecessary requests and, over time, will feel insecure, with imaginable consequences even in his adult life.

Empathic listening is an important way to continue to face the child with respect and attention. Listening is the basis of an educational style that respects the child and recognises him as a person.

I think this behaviour is essential to give the right answers to the real needs of the child. Often the adult interprets the child's behaviour by projecting his needs. This will not allow the construction of effective responses for children and will only cause fear, anger and irritation.

The needs that the newborn expresses through the languages available to him are always important signals that, through the answers he receives or does not receive from the external environment, influence his personality.

Being heard:
- Increases one's self-esteem;
- Stimulates the relationship effectively;
- Establishes emotional relationships.

It is very important to respond to the needs of the child according to the stages of development that he is experiencing. Once again, it will be sufficient to observe and listen to the child to understand that certain needs have changed and that he asks us to grow, to change.

The Author

Bianca Buchal

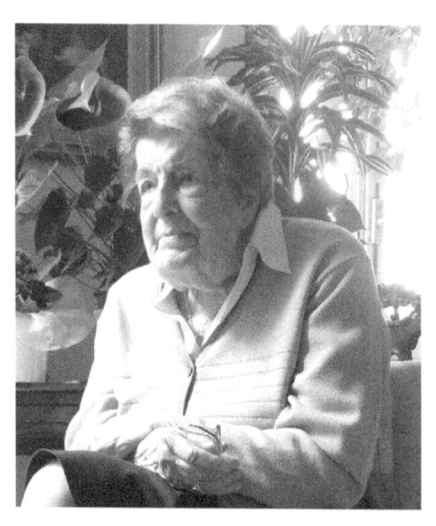

She has been working for decades on birth and has actively participated in multiple associations devoted to this purpose, occupying managerial roles.

For over ten years she has been the Italian delegate for the OMAEP – *Organisation Mondiale des Associations pour l'Education Prénatale* – based in France, she has dedicated her life and has participated in numerous seminars and conferences on the prenatal theme, in various parts of Italy.

She launched an experimental project in order to introduce into schools the theme of *"conscious birth"* with the approval of the Ministry of Health.

She has translated numerous texts and publications on the same subject from French, English and German.

In 2002, she promoted and coordinated a series of conferences on conscious pregnancy sponsored by the City of Milan.

Since a few years, she created a website www.gravidanzaconsapevole.org that she coordinates and keeps alive.

Since 2009 there also is an English version available www.maternityawareness.org.

Printed in France by Amazon
Brétigny-sur-Orge, FR